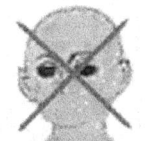
Sexual
Transmission

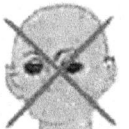
Infected
Mother

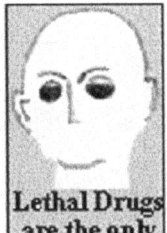
Lethal Drugs
are the only
cause of
AIDS Deaths

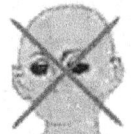
Infected
Needle

Blood
Transfusion

AIDS CARE

AS PER
WORLD HEALTH ORGANISATION'S GUIDELINES
ON TRADITIONAL & NATURAL MEDICINE

by

Dr. Leo Rebello

ND, Ph.D., MD (TNM), D.Sc., FFHom, DHS, MBA, D.Litt., LL.D.

USED FOR SKILLS BUILDING WORKSHOPS
AT UNAIDS CONFERENCES, SINCE 2000.

AIDS CARE

Revised Title

© **Dr. Leo Rebello**

ISBN-13: 978-1495483264
ISBN-10: 1495483266

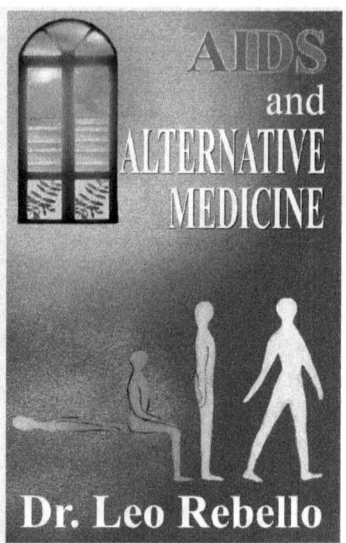

5th Edition, February 2014
of popular book: AIDS and
Alternative Medicine
4ᵗʰ Revised Edition, August 2006
3ʳᵈ Edition, March 2003
2ⁿᵈ Edition, December 2002
1ˢᵗ Edition, June 2000

Book and cover designed by Robin Rebello
Email: actor.robinrebello@gmail.com

Cover depicts that AID$ $CARE becomes AIDS Care
when you turn to Holistic Healing.

This book, based on original research, has educated thousands of 'Persons Living with AIDS' to live healthy with safer, cheaper, reliable and absolutely scientific traditional and natural medicines. You have a 'Right to Know', 'Right to Health', and 'Right to Life' options.

Published by
NATURAL HEALTH CENTRE
28/552, Samata Nagar, Kandivali East, Bombay 400101, India.
Email: prof.leorebello@gmail.com
Website: http://www.healthwisdom.org
Skype id: drleorebello

Printed by CreateSpace

CONTENTS

1st EDITION PREFACE
AIDS REDISCOVERED

Ever since AIDS was 'rediscovered' in 1981, it has threatened the very fabric of society. It was 'rediscovered' by the proponents of Modern Medicine to camouflage its dismal performance in the cause, the course and the cure of major maladies. AIDS (*Oja-kshaya* according to *Ayurveda*) has been in existence ever since man invented fire and started cooking food. Ayurvedic practitioners have managed it by balancing *Tridoshas* – *Vata* (gas), *Pitta* (bile) and *Kapha* (phlegm) and regulating the *Para Oja,* which is the basis of immunological strength.

Left to the practitioners of Alternative Medicine, HIV/AIDS patients can be treated successfully, at fractional cost of the costly allopathic killer drugs like AZT and without their side effects. Similarly, a diet consisting of carrot juice, sweet lime, orange juice, wheat grass, coconut water, fresh buttermilk and curds would put them on their feet by boosting their immune mechanism.

This book prepared for the XIII International Conference on AIDS, Durban, July 2000, talks of age-old wisdom. It explains the concepts of living food as against dead food, laxative and constipating food, acidic and alkaline food and how by proper management of diet, and employing other body cleansing methods, immunity can be built up and toxins thrown out of the body. It outlines other prophylactics so that you need not wait for the elusive and costly AIDS Vaccine. (If Cancer Vaccine has not come after 50 years, there is no hope for AIDS Vaccine).

In here are examples of how immuno-stimulant homeopathic, herbal, biochemic drugs are far more effective than the immuno-suppressant and lethal chemical and costly drugs. How yogic regimen, hydrotherapy, acupressure can give symptomatic relief while building the general immunity and increasing the life span of an AIDS patient. How using meditation, music therapy and other de-stressing techniques, people can be stabilized. In short, here is an Alternative and Total Approach which, if you put into practice, you need not run in circles.

Traditional systems of medicine remain the major source of health care for more than two thirds of the world's population, according to the World Health Organisation (WHO Report 1982). Healing concerns change from illness to health. Traditional systems, which are cheaper, safer, faster, more reliable, can be a vehicle for social, political and economic liberation.

The concept of 'renewed tradition' refers to the use of respected principles of the past, forging new guidelines for action in terms of contemporary needs. **Healing is a shared resource, a right for the ill to request and a responsibility for healers (and state) to deliver.** Therefore, will the World Leaders wake up and stop this obdurate obstinacy and medical hegemony unleashed by proponents of modern medicine and dictated by transnational pharmaceutical lobby, whose only concern remains profits?

May it be noted that over the years, with the onset of modern medicine more people have died due to drugs than the war casualties, pestilence or malnutrition deaths put together. This is unnecessary and has to stop. Let us bring some humanism in medicine. Let us understand the simple truth that 'Health Care is Self Care'.

I invite you to join me and others in removing HIV/AIDS scourge from the face of the earth, like polio, small pox, plague, etc. by following the path of Traditional and Natural Medicine and by changing the focus : From 'Aids Scare' to 'Aids Care'! This is the only way out. The other road leads to Hell.

Whether it is substance abuse, sexual promiscuity or HIV/AIDS, prevention lies in commonsense approaches and treatment in Holistic Healing. I hope this book will change your thinking and your lives. As Alexander Pope opined :

> *The learn'd is happy*
> *nature to explore,*
> *the fool is happy*
> *that he knows no more.*

Dr. Leo Rebello

Bombay, 6th June, 2000

2nd EDITION PREFACE
ALTERNATIVE VIEWPOINT
1st December, 2002

As usual, pharmaceutical mafia's presence was overbearing at the XIII International Aids Conference. But the Durban conference organisers were relatively more open to the alternative viewpoints. My workshop on **Aids and Holistic Healing** was oversubscribed. The manual prepared soon exhausted, leaving a heavy demand for it. I am, therefore, pleased to place in your hands this second revised and enlarged edition.

This book does not conform to the established mafiosi set-pattern of thinking on HIV and AIDS. Nor does it peddle disinformation, disease and death. I implore you to read this book with an open mind and practice what is prescribed therein. It is the wisdom of the yore and it shall not fail you unless you are ostriches who masquerade as 'eminent medical scientists' hopping from one conference to another spreading lies, half-truths and untruths.

Many people who have AIDS don't have the money to buy food, let alone the medications they need. It is necessary that they do not suffer from malnutrition - which is why it is important that patients learn to rediscover their traditional meals and medicines. The 'standard' western diet is very high in toxins. Western medicines likewise are lethal. They do not heal they kill. Western Lifestyle + Western Diet = Western Diseases. The solution to AIDS as also to safety of human beings, development, or world peace lies in oriental wisdom.

The principles of healing are very simple: (a) the body heals itself, (b) there is an inner environment, and (c) treatment should not be worse than the disease. This handy book will tell you more about AIDS and Holistic Health than any other book so far. For wider awareness, any one wishing to sponsor, translate or reprint this comprehensive treatise, in other major languages, is welcome to contact me.

On this World Aids Day, as I release the second revised and enlarged edition of this path-breaking book, I appeal to everyone to throw away blinkers and work for removing AIDS from the face of the earth, following the guidelines prescribed in this master-plan.

3ʳᵈ EDITION PREFACE
AIDS NO MORE
7 March 2003.

AIDS is the greatest myth of our times. Inspite of voluminous evidence which shows that HIV is not AIDS, the myth is kept deliberately going so that the following multi-trillion dollar industries keep prospering:

(a) Latex industry: condom in simple word, even children know its use now. Boys and girls as young as 15, who were earlier afraid of sex, are now experimenting with condoms giving rise to condom ethics, condom culture, condom civilisation, condom protection, all of which is as fragile as the condom itself. There are two types of condoms - male and female. The production, sale and use of female condoms is restricted. After the 'condom accidents' the ever-alert marketing men invented 'double hat' protection, that means using two condoms to be doubly sure! Simple logic you see: if one condom can protect 50% two give 100% protection!

(b) Eventhough HIV testing is unreliable, non-standardized and dangerous, this is a big business. HIV tests include mostly Elisa and Western Blot, which cross-react with over 60 known medical conditions and illnesses. That means they are positively programmed to create scare!

(c) Then there are microbicides, ostensibly to protect the women. Oils, creams, lotions, potions, gels, pessaries and ofcourse other paraphernalia like stimulators, scrubbers, pastes, etc. Presently there is war between chemical microbicides and herbal microbicides for market share. Consumer, as usual, is at the receiving end.

(d) But by far the most lucrative business is the chemical medicines as usual - protease inhibitors, cocktails, anti-retrovirals, HAART or multi-drug regimen, vitamin supplements. Costlier the medicines more effective they are, is the false belief on which the mercenary medical mafia cashes on.

(e) Some one has 'invented' AIDS Counseling. The counselor is as ignorant as the patient. AIDS Counseling includes: telling HIV positive patient to live with it. Further telling him/her that there is no known cure. Scientists are working on Vaccines. Anti-retrovirals are life-savings. They are costly, but if you do not take them you will die and then what will happen to your family? If a patient were to ask about Alternative Medicine, improved nutrition, change in life style, prompt comes the reply they are all dangerous. Beware of the quacks! That in short is AIDS Counseling.

(f) Then there are 'AIDS Advocates' (usually Americans but working in sub-Saharan Africa) promoting the use of lethal chemical drugs and fighting for and on behalf of the poor patients to 'reduce their price', influencing health ministries to underwrite the costs of 'life-saving drugs' and promoting free or subsidised distribution of AIDS drugs, including to pregnant mothers ostensibly to save the unborn. If there is no food to eat, water to drink, clothes to wear, no problem. But you must have medicines, more the better. **They refuse to accept that Nkosi Johnson, an 11-year old boy, died because of harsh treatment - 50 capsules/tablets, injections, three times of day.** A 'single judge' (he is married alright!), in S.Africa decides what the Presidential Panel of Expert International Doctors could not. Human rights concern you see and he thinks he is the great Solomon and the President of South Africa and his panel of experts are fools!

(g) How can we forget the AIDS conferences and AIDS journalists: local, regional, national and international? Big business. The same people, sponsored by the pharmaceutical companies, parroting the same thing without application of mind, running down those who question them, throwing to wind ethics, morals, professionalism, not considering alternative medicine, ideas, experiments, vision or approaches. Very unscientific.

Ever since AIDS was 'rediscovered' in 1981, it has threatened the very fabric of society. It was 'rediscovered' by the proponents of modern medicine to camouflage its dismal performance in the cause, the course and the cure of major maladies.

There is no known cure for HIV/AIDS is the frightening refrain that you get to hear, not only in Sub-Saharan Africa, but also in Asia. **Those who gave you the idea that people have to live with AIDS, also tell you that you have to live with diabetes, with asthma, with epilepsy, with cancers, with muscular dystrophy, with stress and allergies!** It will be my pleasure to remove this wrong notion. If you can give up your old habits, you can also be cured of any malady - physical, mental, emotional or spiritual: druglessly.

Anti-retroviral drugs (ARVs in short) offer no cure for AIDS. US federal health authorities which earlier supported David Ho's "hit hard and early" to control "AIDS epidemic" argument, now realize that it was a hoax. The toxic effects of ARVs include nerve damage, weakened bones, unusual accumulation of fat in the neck and abdomen and drug-induced diabetes. Many people have developed dangerously high levels of cholesterol and other lipids in the blood, raising concern that HIV positive persons might face another epidemic of heart disease.

Indiscriminate use of ARVs to pregnant mothers is fraught with danger. If a cigarette smoking mother can deliver a 'blue baby', if an alcoholic mother can deliver a 'drunk child', if thalidomide can produce 'monster babies', you are unwittingly playing with the future generation, by demanding that the HIV positive mother be given ARVs compulsorily.

AIDS is the consequence of a suppressed immune system, which has been subjected to repeated onslaughts by four factors that build up toxins and deficiencies in the body. These are: antibiotic abuse, recreational drug abuse, anal sex (which causes toxic shock to the receiving partner) and nutritional stress.

Realization is also slowly but surely dawning that the damage caused by the stressed immune system could be reversed by good diet, yogic and other exercises, herbs available readily, acupuncture, homeopathy, proper rest, avoidance of alcohol, drugs, tobacco, proper hygiene, etc. In other words, a person is to be treated as a whole: body, mind and spirit.

Over the years, it has also become obvious that only gay community and those indulging in substance abuse, progressed towards full-blown AIDS. In other words, what I have said in my book AIDS and Alternative Medicine is now being accepted; that the repeated assaults on the body's immune system by the build-up of toxins, nutritional deficiencies, coupled with unnatural living, lead to AIDS. With that the wisdom is dawning that the damage could be reversed without drugs. This new dimension puts to doubt the accepted belief that a virus, HIV, is responsible for causing AIDS.

The HIV tests, *per se*, are being questioned. These tests, we have always maintained, were of dubious merit. Now, after 23 years and ruining precious lives of young people by creating AIDS Scare, it is slowly dawning on the authorities that indiscriminate HIV tests have played havoc with people's lives. Consequently, HIV test is no longer mandatory in many parts of the world. But ignorance once rooted, takes time to be uprooted. Many private hospitals in Bombay still insist on a routine HIV test before admission. And some Governments are making HIV testing mandatory.

There is enough to show that the HIV tests, Elisa and Western Blot, can show false results when there is cross-reactivity with a host of viral and bacterial species. At least 60 different conditions like influenza, herpes simplex, hepatitis, all mycobacterium bacterial species (including leprosy and tuberculosis), malaria, malnutrition and even in pregnancy, persons may be tested positive and falsely labeled as such, ruining their lives and that of their families.

The fact that the HIV test is not specific for the detection of the virus is clearly stated in the literature accompanying the Elisa test kits (from Abbott Laboratories, for instance). In the light of this evidence questions arise about whether bombarding the virus does any good to the body.

Overwhelming research evidence from the fields of AIDS, cancers and heart diseases, points to the dramatic difference in disease prevention, made through access to right nutrition, exercise and changed lifestyle.

Africa is cited as the example of a continent in the throes of AIDS. Health historians say that AIDS there, is a consequence of the depletion of the body's nutrition pool over generations and the destruction of the immune system. As sub-Saharan Africa plunged deeper into the cycle of poverty, malnutrition and civil war, it also suffered epidemics of Ebola, Marburg or Lassa fever that stayed with them for decades. AIDS, they say, is the logical conclusion of this onslaught. The deepening economic crisis of India's poor, likewise, will see more people testing 'HIV positive' due to depleting nutritional status, intestinal fluke, stress, accumulation of various poisons in the body and compromised immunity as a result.

This implies that the poor 'AIDS Victims' of the world, as a whole need more than condoms, sex education and a cocktail therapy of questionable value and we need to look at our age-old Holistic Healing modalities, which are safer, cheaper, faster and more reliable than the lethal cocktails.

In 1976, the World Health Assembly acknowledged the potential value of traditional medicine in expanding health services by calling attention to the manpower reserve constituted by traditional health practitioners (resolution WHA29.72). In the following year, another resolution (WHA30.49) urged countries to utilize their traditional systems of medicine. Yet another resolution was passed in 1978, in which WHO was called upon to develop a comprehensive approach to the subject of medicinal plants (WHA31.33). In 1987, the Fortieth World Health Assembly reaffirmed the main points of the earlier resolutions, as well as related recommendations made at the International Conference on

Primary Health Care, held in Alma-Ata in 1978 (WHA40.33). In 1989, a resolution was passed (WHA42.43) that recalled earlier resolutions on traditional medicine, traditional health practitioners, and traditional remedies and affirmed that together they constitute a comprehensive approach to the utilization of medicinal plants in the health services.

The moot point is inspite of several resolutions of the World Health Assembly, why the WHO is according step motherly treatment to Alternative Medicine? Is it ignorance, corruption or big business that decides? Is WHO a health organisation or 'WHOre' of pharamaceutical companies?

Drugs do not heal, they kill. The only known cause of HIV/AIDS is lethal drugs! The idea of 'People Living With Aids' is nonsense. It is promoted by the medical mafia who peddle disinformation, diseases and death.

Every disease under the sun can be cured by Holistic Healing modalities. The principles of healing are very simple: (a) the body heals itself (b) there is an inner environment (c) treatment should not be worse than the disease.

AIDS is a false alarm. Let us not panic. It is not a dreaded disease as is made out to be. Ayurveda, Nature Cure, Yoga, Homeopathy and other alternative therapies hold tremendous promise in AIDS as also in so-called incurable diseases. Therefore, it is time to halt the wasteful expenditure in dead-end biomedical research and divert those funds to holistic healing modalities. **Even if twenty-five per cent of the total outlay made towards biomedical research is given to alternative systems of medicine, the health graph of the world will show marked improvement.**

'From Aids Scare to Aids Care', 'Aids No More', 'Health Care is Self Care', 'Humanism in Health' and 'Health, Peace and Plenty for All', should be the slogans of the New Millennium.

4th EDITION PREFACE
25 YEARS OF AIDS RACKET

1st July, 2006, World Doctors' Day

The acronym AIDS became a haunting part of the world lexicon in 1981 due to the clever ploy of 'illuminati'. This multi-billion dollar fraud is based on two fabrications: that AIDS is a single disease and that it is caused by the HIV. **HIV+ response means nothing of any relevance to health: it can be triggered by vaccination, malnutrition, measles, influenza, leprosy, glandular fever, hepatitis, syphillis ... : over sixty different conditions.**

CDC or Centre for Disease Control, instead of recognizing its main role to control diseases, created a spectre by reporting five gay men in LA with a rare pneumonia found in patients with failing immune systems (June 5, 1981). To the frustrated researchers of the "war on cancer" program of the United States government, AIDS became a new play game. Institutions for cancer research overnight became institutions for AIDS research and the frustrated cancer researchers became AIDS researchers, transferring to "AIDS science" the idea of viruses as a cause. In May 1983, Human T-Cell leukemia virus was identified in patients with AIDS; later renamed human immunodeficiency virus, or HIV. On December 7, 1995, FDA approved first protease inhibitor, drugs that cripple. On December 30, 1996, Dr. David Ho(ax), who pioneered HIV/AIDS inhibitors was named 'Time Man of the Year' thus proving the Orwellian prophesy. On January 31, 1999 "proof" was released showing that the AIDS virus spread from chimpanzees to people in Africa, when it was the contaminated black blood, sent to Africa, which was the cause. On January 28, 2003, President Bush proposed $15 billion in funding over the next five years for an Emergency Plan for AIDS Relief – this is the second phase to spread AIDS through drugs, as per the well-laid out plan in 'Useless Eaters' document. March 24, 2004, FDA approved an oral HIV test that gives results in 20 minutes. ELISA, Western Blot, CD_4 count, T-Cells and other tests continue being big business. *Ullu bananeka dhanda* (Hindi, meaning business of fooling the world) as one pimp in Bombay rightly commented.

In March 2005, New York City health officials identified several patients infected with a rare strain of highly drug resistant HIV. In other words, drugs have all along been useless. In September 2005 patent for AZT expired; FDA approved the first generic versions so that this carcinogen can be made more affordable, so that more people can be systematically killed. In the meantime, the statisticians at WHO, UNAIDS, World Bank played havoc with cooked up statistics to frighten the world by clubbing deaths due to 60 odd diseases as AIDS. Create scare, sell medicines, weaken people, make them dependent on drugs and rake in profit. That is the kind of nonsense modern medicine is.

Look at this announcement of the Global Health Council, for example: "HIV can be prevented only if there is a reliable and consistent supply of more than 120 commodities, which include HIV test kits, high quality ARV drugs, medicines for treating opportunistic infections and sexually transmitted infections, contraceptives and consumables". Do you need more proof to expose the business agenda of the sickness industry?

For 25 years now the medicine mafia has been fooling the world in the name of HIV/AIDS and for over 50 years in the name of Cancer. In both, viruses and vaccines have not been found and will never be found, because the whole premise of modern medicine of looking at a disease is distorted. It is an affront to human intelligence, that inspite of tremendous growth in ICT, we have been hoodwinked for the last 25 years in the name of HIV/AIDS, defying the logic and stark facts which go to prove that AIDS is a racket.

Since 1981 it is being orchestrated that AIDS is a deadly disease and usually caused by sexual contacts; that HIV is a causative organism which penetrates into helper T-cells of the immune system; that the said virus paralyses the immune system of the human body and destroys the genetic material of T-cells and this damage is permanent. This is total rubbish.

For better explanation refer to Ayurveda, Siddha and Unani chapters of this book, in particular. AIDS is called *Oja-kshaya* in Ayurveda, *Vettai Noi* in Siddha and *Al-Zabool* in Unani. Also, the scientific explanations given by Ayurveda, Siddha, Unani are more foolproof and medicines very effective and affordable as against the Allopathic cheating business.

Dr. Hulda Clark in her book, The Cure for HIV and AIDS, avers that intestinal fluke and benzene weaken the thymus and consequently cannot direct the T-cells to fight and it is not difficult to kill this parasite and all its stages. "Infact", she writes, "the intestinal fluke and all its millions of eggs and microscopic stages can be killed in 6 days with an herbal recipe, or in 2 hours with electricity". She gives over 75 case histories of HIV positive turned negative within 6 weeks with Zapper, in her above book. Ayurvedic, Herbal, Homeopathic, Siddha, Unani medicines too cure "deadly AIDS" within one to three months. As against that, the modern medicine mafia says that you have got to live with the disease and keep taking ART drugs (carcinogens). **So, it is very clear what is more scientific – the modern medicine or traditional and natural medicine.**

The 59th World Health Assembly met in Geneva, 22-27 May 2006 and, *inter alia,* adopted a resolution WHA59.11 to include nutrition as an integral part of the overall response to HIV/AIDS. This is what I have been agitating for, for long. In pursuance of my conviction that Diet plays the most important role in diseases and wellness, I will be once again conducting two capacity building workshops (a) on Nutrition for AIDS and (b) on Yoga for AIDS, at the XVI International AIDS Conference, to be held in Toronto, from 13 to 18 August, 2006 and this book should serve as an ultimate guide to all those who are lost in the AIDS maze.

However, to put an end to the AIDS racket, as also Cancers, Autism and other debilitating diseases, we need to: **(a)** discard the pseudo-science called modern medicine with its faulty paradigms, false research, blatant profit mongering and promotion and pushing of synthetic drugs into our bodies. **(b)** Stop production, sale and distribution of vaccines containing contaminated serum, carcinogens and toxins. Instead give boost to safer Alternative Vaccines. **(c)** Recognise that AIDS is a condition and is not caused by heterosexual sex but by several factors. **(d)** Recognise the adverse role of suppressive treatment, malnourishment, and toxic ART drugs behind AIDS deaths. **(e) Adopt holistic healing methods as outlined in this comprehensive book.**

5th EDITION PREFACE

This 5th Edition of AIDS & Alternative Medicine is being published on popular demand in new title: AIDS CARE.

HIV does not cause AIDS. HIV hypothesis itself is based on unsound science. What causes AIDS is Alcohol and Drugs in homosexuals. Changes in lymphoid organs and adrenal glands are not caused by HIV. Opportunistic diseases in AIDS patients are caused by immuno-suppressive agents, malnutrition and endogenous release of cortisol. Kaposi's sarcoma and lymphoma are also due to drugs. Children's health is compromised by too many lethal drugs in early years, which play havoc on their delicate immunity, and junk food intake as they grow up. The reason why USA is having epidemic of AIDS, Cancer, Diabetes, Heart problems and Obesity.

AIDS in Africa is mainly due to polluted water, malnutrition, vaccines and antibiotics assault instead of providing nutritional food to the poor children of Africa. This, if you don't know, is part of population control pogrom.

On pages 153-154, quotes of several honest, real and reputed authorities are given. If, inspite of that you are not convinced, it is your problem.

In India we have rich tradition of Ayurveda, Yoga, Unani, Siddha and Homeopathy - acronym AYUSH (life). Under the Ministry of Health there is a separate department of AYUSH. In Thailand, where I have addressed high ranking Health Officers, there is a separate Ministry of Traditional Thai Medicine in addition to Ministry of Health. But in India now the onslaught of pseudo-science called evidence-based medicine is growing and more and more fleecing Super-Specialty Hospitals of 'one-disease, one-organ' are spreading. At the same time more and more people are realising that the second invasion of decadent West on India is via drugs, vaccines, junk food, fertilisers, fluoridation of water, chemicals, terminator seeds of Monsanto, colas, pizzas, Big Mac, KFC, etc.

80% Indians, in any case, do not believe in a drug-based sickness care system. We reject the propaganda that for every ill-there is a pill. My candid message: "One can live Healthy Hundred without ills, pills and bills" has brought Wisdom in Health Care. **Bombay, 7 February 2014.**

FROM 'AID$ $CARE' TO 'AIDS CARE'
AN INTRODUCTION

HIV/AIDS is not a deadly disease as is made out. More people die in road accidents, due to malnutrition, substance abuse, with cancers, diabetes, infective hepatitis, malaria, tuberculosis, etc. **And yet, look at some examples of AIDS Scare:**

* They label a patient HIV + and throw up the hands saying there is no known cure.
* They come up with disproportionately blown up statistics and create a false alarm.
* They use highly inaccurate tests for diagnosis of 'HIV Infection'.
* They announce/market hurriedly and/or inadequately tested deleterious drugs, without bothering about future consequences.
* They attack/defame those who say that HIV does not cause AIDS.
* They threaten those who oppose carcinogenic AZT being prescribed freely.
* They create an illusion of bringing out 'Aids Vaccine' forgetting the fact that Cancer vaccine, in spite of half-a-century research and billion of dollars down the drain, has not been possible.
* They claim they are scientists, but refuse to test *veggie vaccines* or *homeopathic vaccines,* which do not pollute the blood stream.
* They distribute condoms indiscriminately along with untested background material, creating sexual promiscuity and exponential rise in HIV/AIDS.
* They circulate pseudo-knowledge, so-called scientific evidence: cry wolf, cry *Eureka* alternately. And create more confusion on HIV/AIDS.
* They suggest separate wards for AIDS patients and enact inhuman laws (like HIV+ cannot marry or bear children) based on ignorance and false premise. They neglect other diseases/deaths because of 'jaundiced vision' of HIV/AIDS. And to keep the myth going they circulate high sounding scientific hogwash.
* They neglect time-tested traditional/natural/herbal medicines and look askance when qualified '*Holistic Healers*' present their scientific evidence or appeal for funds.

* They know that they lie, they know they are wearing sunglasses, they know that their time is out.

* But in the process, they have thrown our planning, priorities, policies out of gear by creating panic – all for a single point agenda, namely, profits.

***Aids* is a false alarm. Let us not panic. It is not a dread disease as is made out to be.** Ayurveda, Nature Cure, Homeopathy and other alternative therapies hold tremendous promise in AIDS as also in so-called incurable diseases. Therefore, it is time to halt the wasteful expenditure in dead-end biomedical research and divert those funds to holistic healing modalities. *Even if twenty-five per cent of the total outlay made towards biomedical research is given to alternative systems of medicine, the health graph of the world will show marked improvement.*

'From Aids Scare to Aids Care', 'Aids No More', 'Health Care is Self Care' and 'Health, Peace and Plenty for All' should be the slogans of the New Millennium.

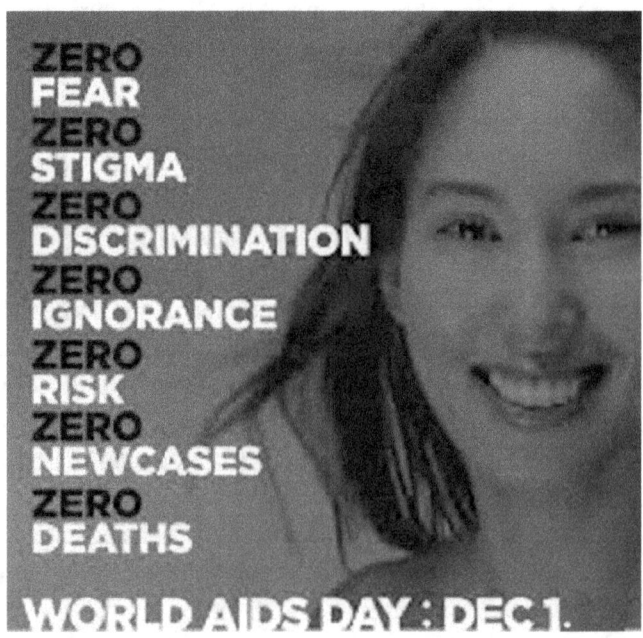

ALTERNATIVE MEDICINE
AN OVERVIEW

Holistic Healing is a descriptive term for a healing philosophy that views a patient as a whole, not at his disease or symptoms. In the course of treatment, a holistic healer may address a client's emotional and spiritual dimensions as well as the nutritional, environmental and life-style factors that may contribute to an illness. Some holistic practitioners combine conventional forms of treatment with natural or alternative treatment.

Holistic Healing is also known as 'Alternative Medicine'. In 1973, the Medical Faculty of the University of Rome convened the first World Congress of Alternative Medicine, and the provisional programme contained no less than 135 different therapies, which could be used as alternatives to the deleterious allopathic system of medicine. Traditional medicine was incorporated in the World Health Organization's programmes in 1976. In 1978, an International Conference on Primary Health Care was held in Alma-Ata, which gave the slogan 'Health for All by the Year 2000'. That lofty goal was not achieved and now we have forgotten it. Though WHO has a separate department to promote traditional and natural systems of medicine, very little is done in that direction since WHO has largely been hijacked by the pharmaceutical mafia.

ALTERNATIVE MEDICINE IS ALSO KNOWN AS :
Traditional medicine (as most of these are practiced from time immemorial);
Complementary medicine (as some allopathic medicine practitioners use them to supplement their medicines to reduce the iatrogenic effect of their drugs);
Holistic medicine (since a patient is looked at as a complete being comprising of physical, mental, social and spiritual dimensions);
Ethno medicine (as these traditional health care systems are closely associated with the life and culture of the masses);
Natural medicine (as these methods of treatment are based on the laws of nature and natural substances are used to treat the patients).
Every country, region or area has its own traditional system of health and

medical care. For the Chinese it is acupuncture; for the French - magnetic healing, for the Germans - heilpraxis, for the British - herbalism; for India - ayurveda; in the Muslim countries, it is unani; in Japan it is shiatsu, and so on.

SALIENT FEATURES OF ALTERNATIVE MEDICINE :
1. Considers the human body as a whole being, that is, the sum total of its physical, mental, social and spiritual dimensions.
2. No side effects.
3. Remedies are based on natural ingredients or they are drugless.
4. Low cost.
5. Simple to prescribe and practice.
6. Preventive and promotive aspects of health are equally cared for.
7. Permanent cure for many so-called incurable and chronic diseases.
8. Faith of the people.

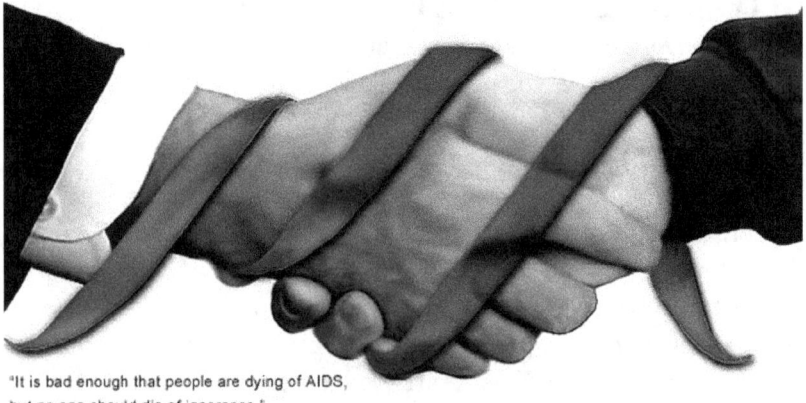

SPREAD THE WORD..
NOT THE VIRUS!
STOP AIDS!

"It is bad enough that people are dying of AIDS, but no one should die of ignorance."

A TO Z OF ALTERNATIVE MEDICINE

A quick look at **Allopathy,** before we proceed to Alternative Medicines, will give us better understanding. Allopathy is also known as 'scientific medicine', 'orthodox medicine' and 'modern medicine' lays emphasis on drugs, drugs and drugs. It offers antibiotics, synthetic vitamins, steroids, chemotherapy, radiation, and immunization all of which are highly dangerous. Its diagnostics methods are not foolproof and 95% of surgeries in allopathic hospitals are unnecessary. Doctors of modern medicine receive their continuing education from Medical Representatives of *(P)harmaceuticals,* and prescribe lethal drugs based on cuts and commission. These inadequately tested and prescribed drugs create more diseases. Allopathy is a 'pseudo science'. It has done severe harm to health and wellbeing of people. As against that see what the 40 odd systems of healing described below have to offer.

Acupuncture/Acupressure : In this age-old Chinese system, the body is divided into 14 meridians and 365 specific points to stimulate, disperse and regulate the flow of vital energy and restore a healthy balance. In acupuncture, needles are inserted at these points, whereas in acupressure only finger pressure is used. Acupoints are also stimulated by a low-frequency electrical current (electro-acupuncture), or with finely tuned laser beams. Some times *moxa* (common mugwort) heat is used over specific points (*moxibustion*), some times needles dipped in homeopathic mother tinctures are inserted (homeo-puncture). In addition to pain relief, acutherapy is used to improve well being and treat acute, chronic and degenerative conditions. Under acupuncture anaesthesia minor/major operations are conducted effortlessly with conscious participation of the patient.

Ayurvedic Medicine : Practiced in India for more than 5000 years, ayurvedic tradition holds that illness is a state of imbalance among the body's systems. These imbalances can be detected through diagnostic procedures like : *Nadi* (pulse), *Mutra* (urine), *Mal* (feaces/stools), *Jeevha* (tongue), *Shabda* (tone clarity), *Sparsh* (touch), *Netra* (eyes), *Akruti* (figure). Nutrition, counseling, massage, natural medications, meditation and other modalities are used to address a broad spectrum of ailments.

Biofeedback : is a practical psychosomatic medicine according to which the autonomic nervous system can be trained. With this, blood pressure can be lowered, cold hands warmed, migraine and epilepsy treated, hemiplegias rehabilitated and deep meditative states induced. Any bodily or mental function that can be monitored can be altered.

Biotesting and Biotherapy : This is a total cleansing process. This therapy helps to eradicate the root cause of diseases by removing the viruses, bacteria, chemicals and toxins stored in the body. A bio-therapist asks the patient to think of his problems and starts the treatment by giving anti-dotes as per the body's requirement. As the anti-dote is placed in the patient's palm, the practitioner starts tapping the thighs of the patient to let the anti-dotes flow in the body. This therapy has shown encouraging results in cases of AIDS, Cancers, Meningitis, Hepatitis, and Malaria and host of other toxic symptoms.

Chromotherapy : Our body is composed of seven colours of the Rainbow, namely : violet, indigo, blue, green, yellow, orange and the red. Thought patterns as also breathing can change the colours in the body. Consequently, the seven colours and sub-colours are used in the treatment of various diseases of the body and the mind. The body synthesizes colours from fruits, vegetables and food eaten. A solarium, colour suncharged water, 12 tissue salts which emanate different colours, are used by experts of Chromotherapy in treatment. It is a fascinating art and science.

Colonics : Using sterilized equipment, filtered water is gently introduced into the rectum, which softens and expels stagnated faecal matter and colon poisons from the large intestine. Colon malfunction can lead to 80% of diseased states. Keep the innards clean and you will be fine throughout your life.

Counseling : This broad category covers a range of practitioners, from career counselors to psychotherapists who treat depression, stress, addiction, and emotional factors. Formats can vary from individual counseling to group therapy. Some therapists may also incorporate bodywork, ritual, energy healing, and other alternative modalities as part of their practice.

Dance therapy : Dance and/or movement therapy uses expressive movement as a therapeutic tool for both personal expression and psychological healing. Practitioners work with people with physical disabilities, substance abuse, sexual abuse cases, eating disorders, and other concerns.

Diet therapy : No matter what name you give to a dis-eased body state, the cause is ever the same! The bottom line or the root cause of any illness, by any name, is simply too much acid tissue waste in your body fluids or your body organs. A body fluid in an alkaline base state is your key to lasting health and eternal youth. Your major five body fluids, *saliva, blood, mucous, lymph and urine,* have the important job of carrying *acid* wastes out of your body. Keep these body tissues and body fluids *alkaline,* to keep our bodies in a constant state of tingling *vibrant health.* Diet therapy therefore concentrates on Alkaline Diet versus Acid Diet, Constipating Diet versus Laxative Diet, Living Diet as against Dead Food, and Perfect Food versus Junk Food. It also considers seasonal food, hot and cold food, and the input and output ratio of food and water intake.

Ear Candling : Primarily used for wax buildup and related hearing problems. Ear candling is also used for ear and sinus infections. Treatment involves placing the narrow end of a specially designed hollow candle at the entry of the ear canal, while the opposite end is lit.

Feng Shui : Ancient Chinese practice of arranging the home or work environment to promote health, happiness and prosperity. Consultants may recommend changes in the surroundings - from color selection to furniture placement, in order to promote a healthy flow of *Chi*, or vital energy.

Flower Remedies : A method of alleviating negative emotional states that may contribute to illness or hinder personal growth. Discovered by Dr. Edward Bach there are thirty-eight remedies, each flower or bud being specific for an emotional state or a personality type. Flower remedies are made from water in which flowers have been dipped and exposed to sunlight for a few hours. Remedies are administered *sub-lingual.*

Gem Therapy : Vibrations from gem-stones can relieve or remove mental and emotional problems – for example, emerald is said to improve memory; red coral gives beneficial results in anemia, lassitude, pain, collapse and general debility; Ruby balances *tridoshas* and is specific for biliousness and blood disorders. Since AIDS spreads through blood, Ruby can be worn on the right hand.

Homeopathy : Founded in 1790, by Dr. Samuel Hahnemann, it is a therapeutic system that uses infinitesimal doses of natural substances - called remedies - to stimulate a person's immune and defense system. A remedy is individually chosen for a sick person based on its capacity to cause, if given in over dose, physical and psychological symptoms similar to those a patient is experiencing. The four cardinal laws of homeopathy are: **(a)** the law of similars **(b)** the law of drug proving **(c)** the principle of potentisation and **(d)** the theory of chronic diseases. Then there is **(e)** the law of direction of cure **(f)** the law of single remedy and **(e)** the law of minimum dose.

Hypnotherapy : A means of bypassing the conscious mind and accessing the sub-conscious, where suppressed, repressed emotions, and forgotten events may remain recorded. Hypnosis may facilitate behavioral, emotional, or attitudinal changes, such as, weight loss, or smoking cessation. It is also used to treat phobias, stress, and as an adjunct in the treatment of illness.

Imagery: Your thinking or imagination can make or mar you. Imagery can boost the immune response, thereby increasing the activity of natural killer cells to identify and eliminate virus-infected cells, other microbes, and tumor cells. Imagery can lower blood pressure, slow the heart rate, alleviate insomnia, relieve stress and anxiety, treat phobias and obesity, and help regulate menstrual cycles. If you can imagine, it can become real.

Iridology : The diagnostic system based on the premise that every organ has a corresponding location within the iris of the eye, which can serve as an indicator of the individual organ's health or disease. Iridology is used particularly when diagnosis achieved through standard methods is unclear.

Iscador Therapy : centres round the extract of the white-berried mistletoe (*viscum album*) plant which grows on a number of host trees. Mistletoe therapy is directed not only against Cancer cells, but it aims to restore the dynamic equilibrium between cells and organism. The earliest declaration over the use of the mistletoe for the healing of Cancer was made by Dr. Rudolf Steiner, the founder of anthroposophy, in 1904 and was introduced into medicine in 1920 by the Lukas Clinic at Arlesheim in Switzerland by Dr. Ita Wegman.

Joviality/or laughter therapy : creates in the body a different chemistry. When you are jovial or when you laugh, you relax, you breathe freely, your digestion improves, movements are easy, coordination better, thinking cordial, memory becomes sharp and vision becomes clear. Joviality, laughter, love leads to vibrant health.

Kirlian Photography : For centuries, mystics, spiritual healers and psychics have been fascinated by the 'auras'- luminous, misty outlines - that surround people, animals, plants and other animate or inanimate objects. Kirlian photography prints auras that reveal people's mental and physical disorders before they display any outward symptoms. Cancers can be diagnosed by modern medicine in later stages and a lot of time is wasted in sub-classifying them while the patient sinks further in health. A good Kirlian photograph in experienced hands can reveal cancer two years before its onset.

Lamaze Method : The purpose of the Lamaze education is to prepare a mother for happy childbirth. This is done by removing fear from her mind and by making her relax and teaching her how to coordinate her breathing, so that childbirth is normal and natural. Based upon Pavlov's principle of conditioned response, the theory is that the brain can be trained to accept and analyze a given stimulus and select a response to it.

Massage : A general term for a range of therapeutic approaches with roots in both eastern and western cultures. It involves the practice of manipulating a person's muscles and other soft tissue with the intent of improving a person's well being or health. Massage can sooth the body, mind and the spirit.

Music Therapy : The rhythm of life as a healing force has been used since ancient times. Making music, dancing to the tune of music, drawing some revealing patterns on paper with colours as music unwinds, breathing in and out in synchronisation, frees the client from submerged feelings and problems. Many people carry unnecessary burdens of the past which, in an enlightened moment, music helps them to unload.

Naturopathy : The oldest health-care system which emphasizes the curative power of nature, treating both acute and chronic illnesses in all age groups. **The three cardinal principles of nature cure are : (a)** healing is within **(b)** there is inner environment and **(c)** treatment should not be worse than the disease. It is a drugless healing. Naturopathy can cure every disease.

Negative Ion : Air molecules are continually being broken down into positively or negatively charged particles. Negative ion concentration is good for health, whereas positive ion concentration is bad. Urban areas, and homes with many electrical gadgets have positive ions. Negative ion therapy helps people to function better by improving their health.

Ohashiatsu : A system of physical techniques, exercise and meditation used to relieve tensions and fatigue and induce a state of harmony and peace. The practitioner first assesses a person's state by feeling the *hara*, the area below the navel. Then, using continuous and flowing movements, the practitioner presses and stretches the body's energy channel, working in unison with the person's breathing.

Prolotherapy uses injections of natural substances, such as, dextrose, glycerin and phenol in order to stimulate the growth of connective tissue and this strengthens weak, damaged joints, cartilage, ligaments, and tendons. This re-constructive therapy is used to treat degenerative arthritis, lower back pain, torn ligaments and cartilage, carpal tunnel syndrome, and other conditions.

Qi is a pre-physical energy existing in air. *T'ai chi* which means great pole or axis is a form of active meditation which helps in tapping the *qi* or *chi* or *prana*. Breathing is faulty in almost 90% people. Due to wrong breathing there is insufficient oxygen in the blood. This leads to hypoxic diseases, like cancers, gangrene, heart attack, stroke, impotence, low vitality, etc.

Radionics and Radiesthesia : Some men and women have the capacity to transmit a steady flow of healing; others, sorcerers, on occasion transmit harm. Inherent within most of us is the ability to switch on to receive healing and to provide it. Radionics and radiesthesia are methods of recapturing and exploiting these largely dormant powers. Radionics is an instrumentally tuned form of distant healing, whereby everybody and every condition can be treated. Radiesthesia has a predictive aspect to it and, as such, its application to prevention presents interesting possibilities.

Reiki is the fine art of tuning the body, mind and the spirit. Practitioners of this ancient healing system use light hand placements to channel healing energies to the recipient. Reiki is commonly used to treat emotional and mental distress as well as chronic and acute physical problems, and to assist the recipient in achieving spiritual focus and clarity. The five principles of Reiki are : Just for today, I will live with gratitude. Just for today, I will not worry. Just for today, I will not be angry. Just for today I will do my work honestly. Just for today, I will love and respect every living being.

Shiatsu : The most widely known form of acupressure. Shiatsu has been used in Japan for more than 1000 years to treat pain and illness and for general health maintenance. Using a series of techniques, practitioners apply rhythmic finger pressure at specific points on the body in order to stimulate *Chi*, or the vital energy.

Silva Mind Control : This technique teaches you how to tap brain-waves as an aid to the development of greater mental discipline. It is a combination of Autosuggestion and Meditation to expand intuition and extrasensory perception.

Tibetan Medicine : Evolved as a synthesis of Tibetan, Chinese, Persian medicine, and Ayurveda. Tibetan remedies include indigenous herbs, fruits, flowers, metallic powders and minerals given in tablet or powder form, and are especially effective in treating rheumatism, asthma, gastritis, diabetes and many neurological disorders.

Unani : Involves the use of plants, herbs and minerals. Known to provide cures for diseases, such as, sinusitis, leucoderma, rheumatism, jaundice and elephantiasis, Unani Tibb or Graeco-Arab medicine is mainly practised in the Indo-Pakistan subcontinent. The basic framework of the four-humour theory of Hippocrates, which presupposed the presence in the body of four humours : blood, phlegm, yellow bile and black bile. Vital force or life-force is called *Ruh* in this system of health care.

Vitamin therapy : A complementary therapy of vitamin usage combined with other treatments to address a range of illnesses and to enhance the functioning of the body system. Assists the immune system in combating chronic fatigue syndrome and HIV/AIDS.

Water therapy : Also known as hydrotherapy, it is a treatment of diseases by means of water in various forms and temperatures. For example, ice massage is given in Parkinson's disease and paralysis, steam for throwing out impurities from the body by opening blocked pores of the skin. In enemas, stomach wash, douches, sitz baths, spinal baths, compresses - cold or warm water is used, both internally and externally. Water is the best cleanser and healer, as 70% body is made of water.

X-ray therapy or X radiation : radiated medicine is used to treat diseases like cancers, tumours, genetic deformities and to nullify radiation effect in the human body. This is not the same as irradiation.

Yoga : It is an eight-fold method of evolving an ordinary man into a super human being. Yoga connects an individual with the universe. It consists of *Asanas* (physical postures), *Pranayam* (breath control), *Kriyas* (cleansing techniques), *Mudras* and *Meditation* (for mind control). Yoga addresses mental and physical problems, while integrating body, mind and the spirit.

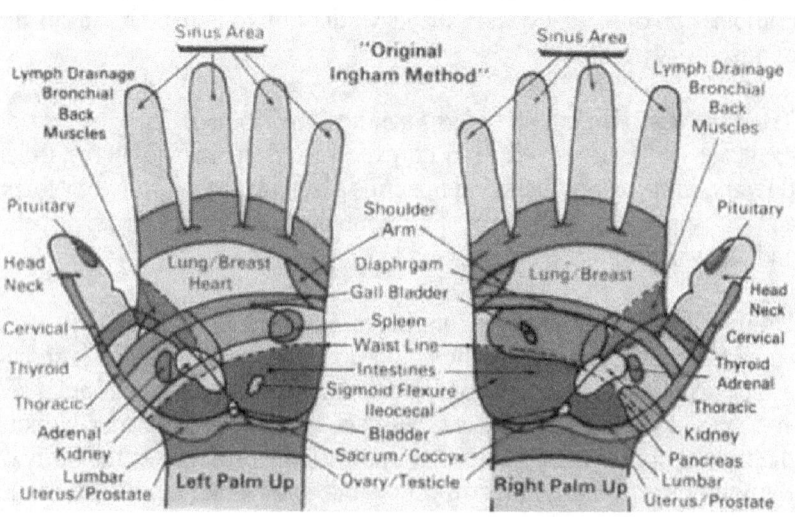

Zone Reflexology is based on the idea that specific points on the feet and hands correspond with organs and tissues throughout the body. With fingers and thumb, the practitioner applies pressure to these points reflected in the feet or hands to treat a wide range of illnesses, as shown in this chart. Reflexologists believe that illnesses show up as tender spots on the reflex areas of affected organs. By pressing the correct points, they treat almost any organ or area of the body. Most parts of the body have corresponding points on each extremity and pressure therapy opens blocked energy channels. For AIDS patients full body massage is contraindicated. But, without hesitation, reflexology or acupressure can be used beneficially.

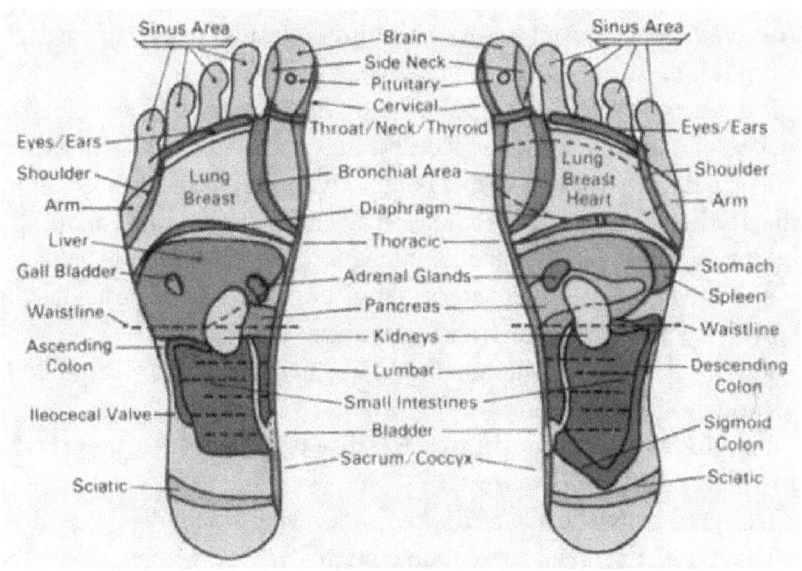

From the description in this chapter, you would note how the Holistic Healing modalities are far superior to Modern Medicine's treatment-oriented chemical approach, which only tackles the human body in parts, not bothering about the mind and spirit aspect. Modern medicine does not also know anything about 'soul sickness'.

NATURE CURE & AIDS

"Man is one and our salvation lies eventually in a mutual sharing of all knowledge" – says Richard Grossinger in 'Planet Medicine'. To that I may add that life is eternal and this intricate human body comes with a guarantee card of 100 years of fault-free service from the finest manufacturer – God. If we suffer unnecessarily and die prematurely, it is because we live unnaturally.

Nature Cure is based on instinct and common sense, and hence, cannot fail.
* It declares that the laws of Nature are immutable and infallible; that sickness is unnecessary and proceeds from violation of the laws of nature;
* That pain is penalty for wrong doing, a warning against transgression; that the body has an in-built defense mechanism consisting of about 120 billion WBCs in 70 kg man, compliments C_1 to C_{17} (special chemicals which break the walls of bacteria, fungi, etc.), hydrochloric acid in the stomach which kills bacteria and antibodies;
* That healing is from within and consequently you alone are responsible for your health;
* **That biomedical changes precede disease and that toxemia is the principal cause of diseases;**
* That cure cannot be obtained without cleansing or removing the cause;
* That body, mind and spirit should be treated as a whole, so that the individual learns to regulate his own life and command his own destiny;
* That in purity lies our power – pure air, water, food, light, environment, thought, purpose and faith.

AIDS is nothing but weak immune system leading to serious breach in the defenses, the vitality of the individual being at its lowest. Due to onslaught of diseases and drugs, AIDS destroys the life of the blood. Even in such a critical condition, however, the body can be encouraged by right living to create its own immunity, manufacture its own antibodies and preserve its integrity without outside help.

The aim of this approach to HIV/AIDS is to balance up the 'poles' again. Ayurveda calls it balancing of *Tridoshas : Vata, Kapha* and *Pitta*. Acupuncture says that to treat a disease we need to clean the meridians and balance the *Yin* and *Yang*. Yoga will say that through *Asanas, Pranayam, Kriyas,* etc. make the body so powerful that the *Vital Force* keeps at its best and flows unhindered through the *Nadis* (Nervous System or Meridians). Natural Healing will enjoin that to remove the debris of food, dead cells, disease taints (*miasms* according to homeopathy), clogging, genetic mutation, take to Alkaline food rather than Acidic, or simply put, avoid constipating or dead food and take plenty of laxative and live food. (See *Diet and Aids* chapter, for details).

Nature Cure does not deny the existence of microbes. But from the nature cure viewpoint, they do not begin the trouble. No infectious disease can be 'caught' until and unless there is a soil for the disease germs to flourish. When we treat by the nature cure method we go back to the cause of the disease instead of just concentrating on the symptoms.

METHODS : There are various methods of living and treatment. ***Return to Nature*** by the regulation of eating, drinking, breathing, bathing, dressing, working, resting, thinking; the moral life, sexual and social activities, on a normal and natural basis. ***Elementary remedies,*** such as, water, air, light, earth-cures and magnetism. ***Chemical remedies,*** such as, scientific food selection and combination, homeopathic medicines, simple herb extracts, and the vito-chemical remedies. Mechanical remedies, such as, physiotherapy, yoga asanas, massage, and osteopathic manipulations. ***Mental and spiritual remedies,*** such as, proper relaxation, normal suggestions, constructive thought, zeroing technique, hypnotism and music therapy. Let us look at some of these natural methods briefly.

1. Fasting : If the body carries a great deal of waste material, one tires very easily and general aches and pains may be felt in any part of the body, most likely along the backbone. Along with this goes a feeling of pessimism and negativism. Our impaired and clogged body mechanism is the payment for the long years of abuse we have forced it to endure.

During fasting, the digestive mechanism of the body is given a rest, the body lives on its own reserves, and old, diseased, cancerous cells are eliminated. What is left constitutes the nucleus, or basis, of a new sound body. Several studies reveal that Cancer cases which went into 'spontaneous remission' were due either to fasting or high fevers (what is known as healing crisis).

The enforced fast undoubtedly has its rejuvenating effect. The cells, tissues and organs, deprived of all unused and precipitated blockade materials, are ready to be replenished anew. This physical rebirth, as it were, might well be a major factor in the physical superiority of the *Hunzakuts*. And it is more than likely that their seasonal fasts tend to keep them humble, friendly, helpful and devotional.

Fasting accomplishes the following changes :
* Vital organs get rest.
* Empties digestive tract and destroys bacteria.
* Gives the eliminative organs a chance to catch up.
* Re-establishes normal physiological chemistry and secretions, thereby regulating digestion and assimilation.
* Promotes absorption of exudates and disused tissues by auto-lysis, whereby tumours and growths subside.
* Restores youthfulness to cells and tissues.
* Permits conservation of nervous energy so that it can be used for repair and regeneration.
* Complexion improves, skin clears up.
* Loose teeth tighten up and bones in fracture heal quicker.
* The heart becomes stronger and the heart pulse more normal.
* The liver becomes smaller, pancreas are toned up and the kidneys get a new lease of life.
* The brain uses ketone from the breakdown of fatty lipids to sustain itself thus saving the glycogen reserves.
* Fasting clears and strengthens the mind and improves functions throughout the body.

2. Colonic Irrigation : Correct functioning of the colon is a necessity for health, for disease can truly begin in the colon. It has been said that colon malfunction can lead to 80% of diseased states.

In health, bowel transit time from eating to defecation is 24 hours or less and bowel movement is at least once daily. In disease, poor digestion, yeast overgrowth, spastic colon, irritable bowel syndrome, chronic constipation and diarrhoea are usually accompanied by auto-intoxication (the re-absorption of soluble wastes into the bloodstream) which places a heavy burden upon the other eliminative organs of the body, the kidneys, the skin and the lungs.

Chronic constipation can lead to further direct complications : diverticulitis, piles, fissures, atonicity, spasticity, prolapsis, colitis and even bowel cancer as well as chronic toxic condition in the rest of the body, like acne and eczema, the cardiovascular system, the nervous system and the liver.

Colonic hydrotherapy is an internal bath that helps cleanse the colon poisons, gas, accumulated faecal matter and mucus deposits. Such techniques were first recorded in 1500 BC, and have been used in traditional and naturopathic medicine since then. Using sterilised equipment, filtered water is gently introduced into the rectum which softens and expels faecal matter and compacted deposits. By improving elimination, response to dietary, homeopathic, herbal, manipulative and other therapies is markedly improved.

3. Hydrotherapy : It is treatment of the diseases by means of water of various forms and temperatures. Water has curative powers. Water exerts beneficial effects on the human body. It equalises circulation, boosts muscular tone and aids digestion and nutrition, tones up the activity of perspiratory glands (in this process eliminates the damaged cells and noxious matter) and aids in removing harmful causes that affect the body.

Water can cure aches and pains, rheumatism, neuritis, auto-intoxication, chronic inflammation, kidney diseases, fevers, haemorrhoids, spasmodic affections of the bowels, high blood pressure, heart weakness, insomnia.

Hydrotherapy is by all means the most powerful and effective of all available therapeutic agents. Besides being free, it is so simple to use water treatment.

4. Yoga Therapy : All of you know that there are life-saving drugs, but how many of you know that there are also life-saving exercises. These exercises are *yogasanas, pranayams and kriyas*. Yoga teaches that a healthy person is a harmoniously integrated unit of body, mind and spirit. Therefore, good health requires a simple, natural diet, exercise in fresh air, a serene and untroubled mind, and a spirit full of awareness that man's deepest and highest self can be recognised as identical with the spirit of God. The law of yoga is the law of life.

If you practice yoga postures, you are strengthening the body. If you control your breathing, you are creating a chemical and emotional balance. If you concentrate your mind in affirmations, you are practicing the power of prayer. But if you synthesize all these, you are entering the most powerful mystery of healing: the basic harmony of life. (See *Yoga Therapy* chapter for illustrations and more details.)

5. Relaxation : Living in an age of anxiety, we are often unconscious of tensions building within us. With normal bodies, why are we depressed, tired, a prey to disease? Because, tension is invisibly draining away our health energies. I describe below, briefly, four techniques of relaxation:

(a) *Shavasana* means corpse-like posture. Lie supine on the ground in a noiseless room, letting all the tight muscles go flaccid, with legs spread-eagled, arms let loose, head tilted to a comfortable side, eyes drooping like closing of petals, play soft music to have hypnotic effect and attain zeroing of thoughts. Best done in the early mornings.

(b) Another method for relaxation is the *Long Swing* : stand legs apart, hands dangling and then turn from left to right and right to left, hands swinging freely and eyes blinking. Do it for as long as you can, say for five to ten minutes and then go and splash your face with cold water. Best done before going to bed, it benefits insomnia.

(c) Relaxation can also be attained in lunch recess, at tea-time and other intervals by first tightening all the muscles, and then releasing them, after a few seconds. While doing this, keep the chest immobile and do diaphragmatic breathing.

(d) There is another simple method: wash your hands, wipe them, then rub them vigorously and gently apply their warmth by covering your face with both your warm hands. Do it thrice and then take deep breaths five to six times.

Just as mental relaxation is conducive to physical relaxation, so also physical relaxation helps relax the mind. Relaxation is a natural tranquiliser, more effective than tranquilising drugs and without their side effects. Relax and healing can begin.

6. Mental Attitude : The attitude of the mind is of great importance in following the natural regimen of living and treatment. The positive mental attitude of faith and equanimity creates positive electromagnetic energies in the body, thus infusing the system with increased vigour and healing power, while the negative, fearful and worrying attitude of mind creates in the system the negative conditions of weakness, lowered resistance and actual paralysis.

Writes **Renee Taylor** in her acclaimed book 'Hunza Health Secrets': "If we foresee trouble, that is what we get. If we envision success, harmony, health and abundance, we experience these conditions in our lives. Since our thoughts are the invisible builders of our destiny, we should be careful about the kind of thoughts we allow to enter our consciousness. If we find negative thoughts intruding, we must throw them out at once and replace them with constructive thoughts. We are either strengthening or weakening our universe each day by the kind of thoughts we entertain. We are also building or destroying our health and vigour in the same way". *Hate attacks are Heart attacks.*

In reshaping the mental attitude from the negative to the positive, counseling plays a very important role. It enables the AIDS/Cancer patient to remove the deep-seated trauma, negative tendencies in the psyche and to enable him/her to undertake self-fulfilling, creative activities. Likewise, teaching the patient to meditate helps, so that deep-seated tensions may be resolved and to release healing energies from within the self. Some therapists use *Creative Visualisation* so that the patient consciously directs healing to deal with diseased cells and tissues.

7. Liver Flush : The liver is the most important detoxifying organ and maintains the equilibrium of the body. The chemical genius of the Liver is basic to the strong beat of your heart, the wide-open channels of your blood vessels, the soundness of your digestion, the sharpness of your brain, and the strength of your muscles. It combats viruses and bacterial poisons and throws them out of the body. It gets rid of dangerous excesses of medicines. This super-chemist also releases energy from food. Your liver is your life.

In Hepatitis B and C, which are on the rise, in AIDS and Cancers and cirrhosis of the liver and patients who have been exposed to a wide variety of environmental toxins or have had to undergo chemotherapy, doing a liver flush once or twice a year is highly beneficial.

To do a liver flush take 8 ounces of distilled water with 8 ounces of apple juice in which is blended 1-4 cloves of garlic, a hunk of fresh ginger and 1-4 tablespoons of olive oil. Take this each morning on an empty stomach for four days in a row. Follow with a cup of tea made with fennel seeds and dandelion root.

It is a good idea to accompany the liver cleansing programme with plenty of green vegetables or warm apple juice. Cayenne pepper should be taken in capsule form or stirred into a little water, at least three times daily. Begin with half teaspoon of cayenne powder.

The best times to do a liver flush are in the spring or summer. It is invaluable for dredging and removing stored toxins and fat accumulated from a sluggish liver throughout the body. It also helps in safely expelling gallstones. You may take advice from an experienced naturopath. Herbs for cleansing the lymph system may include violet leaves, trifolium, burdock, and blue flag. Dandelion, centaury, and wahoo may be used to tone the liver so that waste may be more adequately metabolised. Yogic postures : *Paschim-))* *tanasan, Halasan, Padhastasan, Ardha-Matsyendrasan* help in squeezing the liver and consequently in throwing out the impurities from the liver. (Read *Yoga Therapy* chapter).

8. Osteopathy : "Man is as old as his spine" is a medical axiom, and by that parameter many are physiologically 50 at chronologically 30 years of age. Since the spinal nerves emerging from in-between vertebrae reach out to all the organs in the chest and the abdomen, it is possible to favorably affect the functioning of these organs by manipulation of the spine. In other words, structure governs the function, which means that if we ensure structural integrity, normal functioning will follow. By freeing the impediment on the spinal nerves by osteopathic treatment, glandular and organic malfunctioning is improved.

9. Massage : Massaging is extremely beneficial for various reasons. It tones up the nervous system, influences respiration and nutrition and speeds up elimination of poisonous matter by the skin, lungs, bowels and kidneys. It quickens blood circulation and metabolic processes. Even constipation and hypertension can be cured by proper massaging. However, massage is contraindicated in venereal diseases, leukemia, advanced pregnancies and fungal infections.

CONCLUSION : Many diseases, as per orthodox medicine, are incurable - the common cold, asthma, diabetes, arthritis, cancers and AIDS. Underlying these diseases are several causative factors : psychological, emotional, dietetic, hereditary or environmental. Nature cure can help in most such cases provided the patient is cooperative. All diseases are curable but not all patients, because patients are basically impatient.

AYURVEDA & AIDS

Ayurveda is the comprehensive system of natural health care, about 5000 years old. According to it, everything in the world is composed of the five *bhutas* (elements), viz. *prithvi* (earth), *apa* (water), *teja* (fire), *vayu* (air) and *akasha* (ether). This is the *Panchabhuta* doctrine. The food that we take is also composed of the above five basic elements. Different combinations of these five elements confer upon different foods, different qualities.

Ayurveda believes that food nourishes body, mind and consciousness. Our physical bodies and mental constitutions are characterised by three *gunas* : *Sattva* (potential energy)*, Rajas* (kinetic energy) and *Tamas* (inertia). Food is classified, accordingly. *Sattvic* food is light, healthy food that creates clarity of mind; *Rajasic* food is tempting and increases activity and agitation; whereas, *Tamasic* food is heavy and dull and gives depression, heaviness and many diseases. Hence, our food should change according to the state of mind and body and to suit the changing climate, season and environment.

Like the food, the human body is also composed of five elements. These five elements get modified in the body into seven different entities called *saptadhatus* depending on the food intake. These *dhatus* are *ahara rasa* (food juice), *rakta* (blood), *mamsa* (flesh), *medas* (fat), *asthi* (bones), *majja* (bone marrow), and *sukra* (semen). Only living food, when eaten with joy, is capable of producing *ojas* which is the essence of *saptadhatus.*

According to *Charak Sutra* 17, the seat of *ojas* is the heart and when this energy circulates unhindered throughout the body, we have a healthy system working with clockwork precision. *Para Oja* (the basis of immunological strength) leads to efficient functioning of the sensory, motor and psychic functions, formation and growth of flesh, clear voice, bright complexion and vibrant health.

In Sutra (aphorism) 15, Charak, the great ancient physician, describes three types of disorders of *Ojas*. The local displacement (*oja visrana*), the generalised displacement (*oja vyapat*) and the complete loss (*oja-kshaya*).

Let us compare AIDS and *Oja-kshaya*, for better understanding. Common signs and symptoms of AIDS are : **(a)** constant fevers; **(b)** allergic manifestations like cough, herpes, skin rashes; **(c)** loss of weight (that is why AIDS is also known as thinning sickness); **(d)** night sweating; **(e)** diarrhoeas; **(f)** neurological disorders; **(g)** mental disorders; **(h)** various opportunistic infections due to decreased immunity.

According to Ayurveda, when *Saptadhatus* are affected it leads to *Oja-kshaya*, immune deficiency. For example : **(a)** Fevers are caused due to affected *rasadhatu*; **(b)** skin rashes, viral infections like herpes zoster, liver disorders are due to affected *raktadhatu*; **(c)** weight loss, wasting of muscles is due to depletion in *mansadhatu*; **(d)** excessive sweating leads to depletion of *medadhatu*; **(e)** severe body-aches, joint pains, loss of hair, change in nails are due to affected *asthidhatu*; **(f)** AIDS dementia and other neurological complications are due to affected *majjadhatu*; and **(g)** lapsing into semi conscious or unconscious state in the final stage of AIDS is due to the loss of *shukradhatu*. *So, is AIDS a new disease? Or a new label to what has been described centuries ago by Ayurveda so scientifically?* Whether it is AIDS, Cancer, Diabetes, or any other disease, the entire edifice of modern medicine is based on fake premise.

According to modern medicine, HIV infection causes progressive immune depletion. It could well be the other way round. Immune depletion could lead to the HIV infection, as body by nature prevents itself from the attacks of several diseases and viruses. As such, HIV alone will not lead to AIDS. Several co-factors are essential for it.

The body's immune system is complex; it is always active and vigilant. Viruses invade mainly the brain, testes, ovaries and the liver. In a 70 kg man there are approximately 120 billion WBCs. The WBCs in the blood perform the major role. Majority of them are phagocytes. Another set of WBCs called lymphocytes make the phagocytes active. They are of two types: the B cells and the T cells. The thymus (located under the top of your breast bone, just below the thyroid gland) is essential to the maturation of the T cells, which live up to five years. These cells are important in the body's cellular immune response. **In other words AIDS is the condition of the weakened thymus.** (For enlarged thymus, allopaths used thymus irradiation, which increased thyroid cancer. Likewise, now they are freely prescribing AZT, a hurriedly withdrawn carcinogen, as the be-all and end-all for HIV/AIDS. So much for their wisdom!).

In terms of Ayurvedic theory : unless there is an inbalance in *Vata, Pitta* and *Kapha* (the three humours), the disease cannot settle in. *Vata* is for movement, *Pitta* is for restoring metabolic activity at digestive level and cellular level and *Kapha* is for balancing cold, strength and overall defence mechanism. To obtain their equilibrium, the *Panchakarma Theory* is described. ***Panchakarma is a scientific theory of detoxification.*** It consists of five actions, namely, *Vaman* (vomiting), *Virechan* (medicated purgation) *Basti* (cleaning the bowels with medicated enemas), *Nasya* (medication through nasal route), *Rakta mokshan* (blood-letting to activate formation of new and healthy blood). This is the basic mode of treatment in Ayurveda. It facilitates faster action of medicines.

Ayurveda treats AIDS by removing the impurities from the cells, the acid from the blood, which is due to the predominance of bile. It prescribes *rasayanas* to purify and re-vitalise the cells. *Rasayanas* are the essence of fruits and herbs brought together to build the molecules, thereby balancing the body. ***Some powerful rasayanas are :*** Indian gooseberry (called *amla*), *guggul* (*balsamodendron mukul*) and winter cherry or *ashwagandha* (*withania somnifera*). They rejuvenate the body. Among them *gotu-kola* (*hydrocotyle asiatica*) and *ginseng* are specifics for *Vata*. Aloe vera, comfrey root, and saffron for *Pitta*. Elecampane (*inula helenium*) and honey are specifics for *Kapha*.

In India, we have many rasayanas. *Chyawanprash*, for example, which contains 26 ingredients in honey/ghee base, is readily available. It is the best tonic for all ages and specific for anemia and other blood disorders. Honey is considered the *shukra*, or purest essence, of the plant world. Likewise, Dr. Balraj Maharishi, an acknowledged master of Ayurveda, has blended *Amrit Kalash* (literally, vessel of immortality), a complex herb and fruit mixture containing, among others, following rasayanas : amla, licorice, sandalwood, honey, ghee, Indian gall nut, butterfly pea, heart-leaved moonseed, wild Indian pepper, elephant creeper, aloe wood and Indian pennywort. *Amrit Kalash* comes in two preparations : a small herbal pill and a sweet jam-like paste.

There are ayurvedic preparations *Immuno-QR* or *Tabaid* which kill the virus and improve the body's immune system. But these medicines *per se* will not work unless the patient observes a strict diet of no alcohol, no meats, no fermented foods. A patient may have to take this immuno-restorative medicine for six to eight months till the lymphocyte count increases, which according to me is an unduly long period. For, in terms of applied nutrition, through proper food selection one could be well on the way towards a healthier blood stream within so short a time as 90 days.

Some other Ayurvedic medicines useful in HIV/AIDS are : *Tapyadi Loha Vati* (health restorative tablet); *Raktashodhak Vati* (for eczema and other skin diseases); *Sukshma Triphala Tablet* (an antibiotic, antiviral); *Shatavari Kalpa and Ashvagandha* (as a general tonic and for hyperacidity); *Dadimavaleha* (a syrup that helps in diarrhoea, dysentery and acidity); *Vasosin Syrup* (indicated in asthma, tuberculosis); *Kanchanar Guggul* (for tumours); *Arogyavardhini tablets* (in ascites, liver dysfunction, recurrent fevers); *Kamadugha tablets* (in herpes, hyperpyrexia, hyperacidity); *Sitopaladi Churna* (tuberculosis, anorexia, pyrexia).

Ayurvedic drugs are easily available. A majority of the drugs of vegetable, mineral or animal origin are available in a kitchen, or in a grocer's shop. The methods of preparation are also simple. They are also less expensive compared to drugs used in modern medicine and without dangerous side effects.

SIDDHA & AIDS

Siddha medicines are supposed to be *Adi Sanatan*; that is, 5000 BC. This science was imparted by Lord Shiva to Parvati (*Adi Shakti*). Parvati gave it to Nandi and Nandi passed it on to sage Agasthiar, who hailed from South India. Therefore, Siddha texts are in Tamil. Many things are common in Ayurveda and Siddha, for example, the three *doshas* : *watam* (gas), *pittam* (bile) and *kapham* (phlegm). *Watam* controls the nervous actions, such as, movement, sensation, etc. *Pitham* controls the digestion, assimilation, warmth, etc. and *Kapham* controls stability according to Siddha. When their equilibrium is upset, disease sets in, which is what even Ayurveda says. Various seasonal changes too affect the body.

Sidhars (Siddha practitioners), like *Vaidyas* (Ayurvedic physicians), also consider *Panch Bhutas* (five elements – see Ayurveda chapter), and *Sapta Dhatus* (seven tissues): *Rasa* (lymph), *Kurudi* (blood), *Tasai* (muscle), *Kozhuppu* (adipose tissue), *Elumbu* (bone), *Majjai* (marrow) and *Suklam* (hormones) in diagnosing and treatment. **Sidha vaidyas too diagnose the disease by following methods :** *Nadi* (pulse), *Mutra* (urine), *Mal* (feaces/stools), *Jeevha* (tongue), *Shabd*a (tone clarity), *Sparsh* (touch), *Netra* (eyes), *Akruti* (figure).

Siddha Medicines are prepared out of precious stones and metals by grinding and burning *(Bhasmas)*. The more they are ground or burnt the more they are potent. **AIDS was called *Vettai Noi* in olden times.** The syndrome was classified into 21 types, caused due to wrong diet, excessive and unnatural sex, leading to imbalance in *Ojas shakti*.

Siddha medicines for AIDS are: *Ayavir chenduram, Idivallathi, Thetankottayleham, Eladi churnam, Amukkar churnam, Kashuri mathirai, Velliparpam, Nandukkaiparpam, Imburleham, Nandi mezhugu, Inji leham and Mahavallathi leham etc.*

According to Dr. A.G. Ganapathy, Dr. V.S. Kanaga Sundaram, the herbs recommended for effective treatment of AIDS are:

(1) *Arugam pul (cynodon dactylon)* – the herb acts as emollient, astringent, diuretic and styptic and is widely used to cure phlegmatic respiratory affections, epilepsy, sleeplessness, liver cirrhosis, ulcerated wounds, etc.

(2) *Karasalanganni (eclipta Alba)* because of regenerative effect of this herb, it is given in liver, spleen and bone marrow disorders. The herb contains sterols, sulphur, glucosides, phenols, tannic and sapomine.

(3) *Musu musukkai (mukai scavrilia)* is mainly used to cure respiratory problems, chest pain, asthmatic condition.

(4) *Thooduvalli (solanum trilobatum)* – purifies and tones up metabolic activity leading to increase in body weight, builds muscle mass and increases libido. Along with *Eclipta Alba*, this herb too is used in *Kaya kalpa.*

(5) *Jeeragam (cuminium cyminum)* this carminative and astringent herb treats dysentery, tuberculosis, and also disintegrates renal stones.

Dr. V. Kalidas outlines the following as supportive medicines for AIDS:-
For purification of blood – *gandhaka rasayanam, parangipattai churnam* and *palakarai parpam.*
For reducing fever – *linga chendooram, gowri chinthamani, thrikadagu choornam, vatha, pitha* and *kapha kudineer.*
For persistent diarrhea – *thair sundi choornam, kavika choornam* and *amaiodu parpam.*
For revitalizing and rejuvenating the weakened immune system of the body – *orilai thamarai karpam, serankottai lehyam, thetran kottai lehyam, amukkira (ashwa gandhi).*
Antiviral drugs of Siddha are *rasagandhi mezhagu, murukkanvithu* and *edi vallathy mezhagu.*
For restoring the disturbed mind – *vallarai (centella asiatica).*

Dr. Ananda Kumar outlines the following Siddha treatment for AIDS:-
Herbal preparations – *serankottai ney, mahavallathy lehyam, parangi rasayanam.*

Herbo-mineral preparations – *gandhaka parpam, gandhaka rasayanam.*

Herbo-mercuric preparations – *idivallady mezhagu, poorna chandrodayam.*

According to Dr. S.Raja Lakshmi and Dr. G. Veluchamy, the Kalpa drugs in AIDS are:-
To Rejuvenate the System: Pon Seendhil (yellow moon creeper); *Pey Churai* (bitter bottle gourd); *Sarkarai Vembu* (scoparia dulcis); *Karanchitra moolam* (plumbaga capensis); *Kuruchit agathi* (sesbania grandiflora, black variety); *Karu Nelli* (black gooseberry); *Nagathali* (opuntie dillenii); *Karu Maruthu* (terminalia tomentosa); *Pey Kadali* (cicer aretinum, wild variety).

To Tone the System: Senkottai (semicarpus anacardium); *Pon Kaiyan* (eclipta plant bearing yellow flowers); *Pon ummathai* (datura plant bearing yellow flower); *Thillai* (excoecaria agallocha).

*Capable of prolonging life: Sarkarai Vembu (*scorpia duclis); *Kodi Nelli* (Indian gooseberry – creeper variety); *Azhu kanni* (Indian weeping tree) and *Tholuganni* (telegraph plant).

Nervine Tonic: Nilappanai (curculigo orchiodes); *Kattu Jadikkai* (myristica malbarica); *Vetrilai Kasthuri* (hibiscus abelmoschus); *Etti -* Strychnus Nux Vomica; *Neer Brahmi* (bacopa moneri), *Vishnu Kranthi* (evolvulus alsionoides) and *Sangu Puspi* (clitoria ternatea).

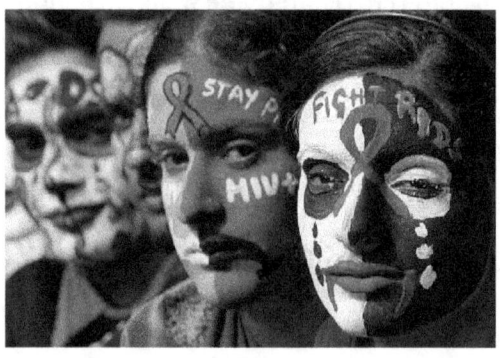

UNANI & AIDS

From 1981 to 1986, HIV was called LAV, HTLV – I, II & III - different names given by different researchers. To "standardize", the International Committee on Virus Nomenclature decided in 1986 that it should be called HIV or Human Immuno Deficiency Virus, and it was further labeled that HIV caused AIDS. **Thus, was born the myth HIV=AIDS=Death, which is totally wrong.**

The word virus in Latin means poison. These viruses being very, very small in size can be seen only under electronic microscope having high resolution. The so-called AIDS virus measures 100nm [1 nm = 1 millionth of a millimeter (mm)] in diameter and 230 million viruses can fit in one full stop. So, how can you identify which of the trillions of viruses, many of which have not even been identified (like HIV has not been identified) that it is HIV and that such a tiny-tiny thing can weaken the powerful body? In other words, as Louis Pasteur himself said on his death-bed, "The germ is nothing; the terrain is everything".

Unani System of Medicine (3000 BC) is one of the ancient medical systems like Ayurveda and Siddha. It originated in Greece and Arabs and Persians further developed it. There are hundreds of colleges in Asia propagating Unani system of medicine and there is a department of Unani Medicine, under the Ministry of Health and Family Welfare, Government of India, which undertakes scientific research in this branch of medicine.

To Unani physicians AIDS is not a new deadly disease. AIDS is called *Al-Zabool* in old medical literature and Unani medicines help AIDS patients to maintain health, reduce infections, increase resistance power, improve quality of life and regain confidence.

Unani Scholar Hakeem Kabiruddin records in his recognized text *"Sareh Asbab"* that excessive loss of *Akhlate Arva* (humours) and *Mani* (semen) etc. weaken the human body. In such a weakened condition, *Azsama Ghariba Khabisa* (viral and other infections) strikes the human body leading to abnormal *Hararate Ghariziya*. This leads to destruction of bodily fluids and melting of the human body, ending in loss of energy and fluid, skin and hair losing their shine, body emitting peculiar odour, etc. This peculiar body odour is found in chronic Acidity, Cancers, Diabetes, Tuberculosis, and AIDS.

Al-Zabool **powder for AIDS contains (each 5 gm):**
Cassia angustifolia (Indian senna) 0.9 gm
Smilax China 1.1 gm
Bambusa arundinacea Retz (the common bamboo) 0.7 gm
Tinospora Cordifolia (Indian quinine or giloe) 1.4 gm
Fumeria (pitpara) 0.9 gm

Al-Zabool is a 100% pure herbal medicine, which effectively stimulates the immune system, increases appetite and strength, thereby improving the quality of life. It is a non-toxic formulation and free from steroids or toxic heavy metals. **AIDS patients using *Al-Zabool* powder have shown following results:**

Persistant increase in CD_4 Lymphocytes count. Increase of haemoglobin. Increase in appetite. Weight gain. Complete regression of opportunistic infections. No side effects even after prolonged use. Feeling of well-being. The minimum duration of treatment (which may vary from person to person) is six months and Rs.5000 (approx.US$100) only inclusive of all taxes, postage, etc. Now compare that with the prices of anti-retrovirals and their side effects.

Alcohol, Nicotine and Tobacco produce severe suppression of the body defense (immune) system and these products interfere with the normal functioning of helper T cells. Like the police issue a red alert against a dangerous terrorist, the body too issues a red alert to the Thymus for regrouping of warrior cells. It is all so meticulously organized. But when the defense system itself is suppressed, the disease multiplies. Anti-retrovirals and other drugs numb the body's immune mechanism and consequently, as I have said time and again, is the ONLY known cause for AIDS.

HERBS & AIDS

The purpose of herbal medicine is to assist the recuperative processes in the body, as they re-establish the physiological balance of health. In herbal medicine, practically all parts of a plant may be used, such as, root, rhizome, stem, leaf, flower, fruit and seed or tissues, bark and wood, or gums and resins. Whole small herbs are used in infusion, or made into tea, others are used as decoction. Other preparations include tinctures, often one part of the herb in five parts of diluted alcohol, or liquid extracts, tablets, powders, lotions, suppositories and inhalants.

Until the beginning of modern science and chemistry, almost all medicines were herbs. Herbal remedies were first systematised in India, China, Greece and Italy. Herbs are natural medicines that contain a variety of biologically active ingredients and are used to successfully treat allergies, bacterial and viral infections, chronic fatigue, immune disorders, cuts and burns, tumours, skin disorders and host of other diseases. Herbs are also used as relaxants, stimulants or as aphrodisiacs. As more and more bacterial infections are becoming resistant to antibiotics, the west is once again turning to herbs.

Herbs are generally safer and gentler than prescription drugs, and often more effective. But certain herbs are toxic and self-medication may prove counter productive.

"In AIDS the waiting period is 2-5 years before resistance breaks down completely", opine so-called AIDS experts. But as Herbologists or Holistic Healers would tell you, death is caused not by destructive virulence but by a lack or loss of the body's defenses, a failure of the regenerative mechanisms; a disease the patient might easily have overcome under normal circumstances.

Herbologists believe that the following herbs can combat AIDS and other viral diseases : *Echinacea* purpurea and angustifolia (purple corn flower), *Hypericum perforatum* (St.John's wort), *Allium sativum* (garlic), *Cochlearia armoracia* (horse radish), *Lycopus europeous* (bugle weed), *Tusilago petasistes* (butterbur), *Mangiera indica* (mango leaves), *Opium* (papaver somniferum), *Bear's garlic* (ramsons) and *Usnea* (containing lichen acid).

Echinacea was used extensively by all herbologists and homeopaths as a curative value in syphilis in all stages. Herbologists have found it as a useful remedy in AIDS with other vitalising herbs like **Alfalfa.** With these medicines in combination, used for about six months, the blood will be free from AIDS. Five drops of Echinacea sublingually, or 10 drops in warm water, three times a day (tds), followed half-an-hour later by a table spoon of Alfalfa. Both these medicines are easily available in herbal as well as homeopathic shops. It is also used in gonorrhoea with very good results.

According to Father Muller, Echinacea is an antidote to all kinds of poisons, viruses and toxins, and thereby cures diseases caused by them. In gangrene of all forms, it surpasses all other known remedies. It acts as an antidote to malaria and is also used in typhoid, diarrhoea, dysentery, cholera infantum, chronic and foetid bronchitis. Boils, carbuncles and affections of glands, psoriasis, lichen planus and other forms of skin diseases respond to it effectively. For native Americans, Echinacea is a sacred plant. Echinacea has the ability to reinforce the body's defense mechanism. It is a remarkable plant to activate the immune system and is a great aid to the body's resistance to micro-organisms.

Hypericum perforatum (St. John's wort) is a great anti-viral remedy containing hypericin. The juice of this plant is toxic. However, in homeopathic mother tincture or in 6x dilution it is safe and effective. It has been used by herbologists and homeopathic practitioners for over 150 years. American herbologists use the tincture of this plant, prepared on homeopathic principles for treatment of AIDS with other supplementary herbal preparations and nourishing diet. Hypericum is anti tetanus.

Mango leaves (Mangifera indica) : Mango leaves have anti-viral properties (isomangifern and managfern) which are very effective against type 1 herpes simplex virus (HSV–1). The mother tincture can be used successfully against AIDS virus in conjunction with other herbs indicated in this chapter.

Allium ursinum (Bear's garlic) : This has a distinct pungent smell, it has considerably more sulphur content than the common garlic. It acts on the skin, bones, bronchial tubes. Bear's garlic can be eaten fresh, in salads. For therapy it can be used in mother tincture. It is also used in blood pressure, strokes, paralysis. It is a tonic herb, it has great effect on hardening arteries. On the whole the herbologists have found the tincture of this plant as anti-viral agent for AIDS in combination with other herbs.

Butterbur (Tusilago petasites) : A very effective antiviral remedy. Must be used only in 6x potency tincture and not lower than 2x potency in dilution. This remedy attacks tumours, growths, and all other pathological cell changes, very effectively. It is a strong medicine. Butterbur reduces sensitivity to pain. Apart from a good slow acting remedy for AIDS it is also a good remedy for asthma, painful menstruation and as an analgesic.

Horse Radish (Cochlearia armoracia) : Dr. William Boericke in his outstanding Pocket Materia Medica records that horse radish raises the vital force and now it has been established that it can be a very important remedy in AIDS. Horse radish has regenerative effect on cases of dysbacteria and helps to overcome functional disorders of the pancreas. A seasoning herb, with antibiotic properties, mother tincture of horse radish can be used in AIDS without any problem.

Lycopeus europaeus (Bugle weed) : Indian herbologists have used it for centuries in advanced and incurable syphilis, including syphilis of the brain, it being a great anti-viral remedy. It also works wonders in palpitation, being a tranquiliser, and in hyperthyroidism. Lycopeus mother tincture is harmless and can be taken 10 drops three times a day. *AIDS being an extension of STD, it can be used as an intercurrent remedy in its treatment.*

Opium (Papver somini-ferum) : Opium is used by French and British Homeopaths in potent form and by herbalists for the treatment of AIDS. Most of them use it in 6x dilution. The effects of opium are shown in the insensibility of the nervous system, the depression, drowsy, stupor, painlessness and torpor, the general sluggishness and lack of vital reaction which constitute the main indications of the drug when used herbally or homeopathically.

For secondary infections, particularly thrush, two tablets of dried golden seal root are recommended twice a day. One to three garlic capsules a day are also very effective. For bowel disorders, about 20 drops of golden seal, in liquid form, should be taken three times a day between meals. Acidophilus is also believed to be effective against thrush and bowel infections. Take ¼ teaspoon of Superdophilus twice a day between meals. Upto three garlic capsules a day might also be prescribed.

According to the preliminary reports on studies done in Thailand and Japan, **Orchids** could prove to be the wonder drug for AIDS. Orchids have long been used as an anti-cancer drug and an aphrodisiac. As a result, large-scale piracy started and the international union of flora and fauna had to intervene to ban the collection of orchids from the wilds. Orchids are grown abundantly in Sikkim, North Bengal, the North East of India, etc.

Finally, we have **Neem** (scientific name *Azadirachta indica*) - nature's panacea for all ills. It is a powerful blood purifier and detoxifier, an antiseptic, antipyretic, anthelmintic and has curative uses in jaundice, dysmenorrhoea, psoriasis, urticaria, pruritus and several skin disorders. However, this 'free tree' given by God to save man has been usurped by the WTO and IPR regimes in the form of patents, patenting in the process greed and monopoly when millions are dying due to penury. It is, therefore, necessary that each one of us goes back to Nature, respects it, avoids tinkering with it for selfish gains.

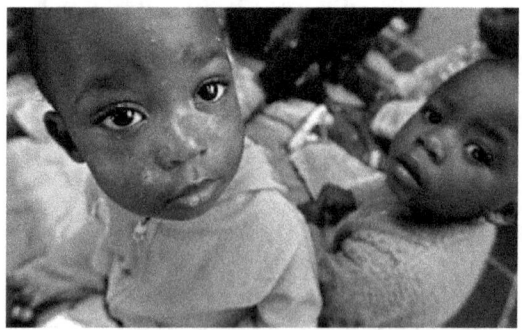

**DON'T KILL OUR AFRICAN CHILDREN.
GIVE THEM NATURAL FOOD, NOT DRUGS.**

HOMEOPATHY & AIDS

AIDS is caused, it is falsely touted, by a virus which spreads through the parenteral route : through infected needles, blood transfusions with infected blood; sexual transmissions; transplacental route : from an infected mother to her foetus. It is further propagated that the damage that the HIV can cause to the immune system can leave the body prey to infections of the lungs, skin, nervous and digestive systems and cancers. "Since a very small number of those with HIV get AIDS, it is thought that a number of other important factors make particular individuals more susceptible".

In Homeopathy, or for that matter in all holistic healing modalities, we look at the patient as a whole. No two patients are alike; even two Siamese twins are not identical. The immune response to disease is a state or a phenomenon, not a mechanism; it has no set location in the body, it is scattered throughout the body and is closely associated with the vital organs in general and with the nervous and endocrine systems in particular. The homeopathic extension of this understanding is that it is also, therefore, reflected in the personality traits and temperaments. Thus, constitutional homeopathic treatment has a distinct role to play in chronic diseases like AIDS. *Sulphur, Syphilinum and Tuberculinum are the three constitutional medicines that emerge in HIV/AIDS cases.* Homeopathy for drainage, immunity and for removing inherited taints is invaluable.

It is said that the HIV+ person may get any one or more of the following complications as the disease takes its toll: diarrhoea, fever, chronic cough, pruritic dermatitis, apthous stomatitis, lymphadenopathy, oral candidiasis, genital ulcers/warts, herpes zoster, chicken pox, pleural effusion, bilateral parotitis, weight loss, Kaposi's sarcoma, pneumonia, and each of these are to be managed properly.

Listed below are some of the Homeopathic Remedies vis-à-vis clinical manifestations :
Diarrhoea : Ars Alb., Calc. Phos., Cinchona Off., Merc Sol., *Phosphorus.*

Fever : Ars Alb., *Phosphorus.*
Cough : Kali Carb., *Phosphorus,* Pulsatilla, Silicea, Rhus Tox.
Pruritic Dermatitis : Rhus Tox., Natrum Mur., Graphitis, *Phosphorus.*
Apthous Stomatitis : Nitric Acid, Merc Sol., *Phosphorus.*
Lymphadenopathy : *Phosphorus,* Natrum Mur., Tuberculinum.
Oral Candidiasis : Borax, Hydrastis, Merc Sol.
Genital Ulcers/Warts : Lycopodium, Syphilinum, Thuja, *Phosphorus,* Kali Bich, Acid Phos.
Herpes Zoster/Chicken Pox : Rhus Tox., Hepar Sulph., Calc. Phos.
Pleural Effusion : Ars Alb., Kali Carb., *Phosphorus.*
Bilateral Parotitis : Calc. Iod.

For AIDS-associated malignancies like Kaposi's sarcoma (a rare malignant tumor of the blood vessels), non-Hodgkins lymphomas (lymphatic tumors), and carcinomas of the rectum and tongue the following homeopathic medicines may be tried :

Kaposi's Sarcoma : Kali Arsenicum, Acetic Acid.
Lymphatic Tumors : Hoang, Iodum, Arsenic Iodide, *Phosphorus.*
Cancer of the Mouth and Tongue : Fuligo Ligni, Galium Aparine, Kali Cyanatum, Sempervivum Tectorum.
Cancer of the Stomach : Condurango, Arsenicum Album, *Phosphorus,* Kreosote, Cadmium Sulph, Geranium.
Cancer of the Rectum : Ruta Graveolens, Kali Cyanatum, Hydrastis.
Cancer of the Vagina : Kreosotum.
Leukaemia : Benzenum, Lycopodium.

Based on the clinical experience of over 4 years, at the Regional Research Institute, at Bombay, under the Central Council of Research in Homoeopathy, Delhi, the observations noted during treatment of HIV carriers were as under :-

Diarrhoea in AIDS - period varied from 2 days to 2 months. Frequency of stools 4 to 12 per day. Stools - watery, with mucus or blood and mucus, associated with pain in abdomen, fever and oral ulcers. Remedies found useful - Arsenic Alb, Cinchona off., Merc. Sol., Nux Vomica, Silicea,

Calcarea Phos, Lycopodium, Natrum Mur, Phosphorus. Treatment duration
: 2 to 10 days.

Fever in AIDS – Lasting from 2 days to 2 months and varying from 99°F to
103°F, associated with cough, diarrhoea, anorexia, oral ulcers,
lymphadenopathy. Remedies found useful - Ars Alb., Badiaga, Natrum Mur,
Bryonia, Cuprum Ars, Phosphorus. Treatment duration - 2 to 10 days.

Chronic Cough – may last from 15 days to 2 months. Type of cough -
dry, productive or non-productive. Nocturnal. Associated with chest pain,
fever, sore throat, breathlessness, pleural effusion. More marked with history
of Koch's. Remedies found useful - Antim Tart, Baryta Carb, Bryonia,
Calc Phos., Hepar Sulph, Kali Carb, Natrum Sulph, Pulsatilla, Phosphorus,
Rhus tox, Silicea. Treatment duration -7 to 15 days.

Pruritic Dermatitis – Ranging from 3 days to 3 months. Area of distribution
– generalised, extremities, face, chest and axilla. Type of lesions – macular,
pappular, maculo-pappular, vesico-pustular, boils. Mostly dry, sometimes
watery or with blood and pus oozing. Remedies found useful – Graphites,
Rhus tox, Natrum Mur, Staphysagria, Petroleum, Syphillinum, Silicea,
Sulphur, Hepar Sulph, Phosphorus. Treatment duration – 7 to 10 days.

Aphthae (mouth ulcers/thrush) – Ranging from 2 days to 15 days. Recurrent.
Superficial, deep, painful and with Fetor Oris. Remedies found effective -
Borax, Nitric Acid, Merc Sol, Silicea. Treatment duration - 7 to 15 days.

Lymphadenopathy (any disease of the lymph nodes in which glands get
swollen or fill with water/liquid). Lasting from 4 days to 3 months. Areas
of involvement - axillary, cervical, inguinal, bilateral, unilateral. Remedies
found effective - Badiaga, Lycopodium, Natrum Mur, Silicea, Calcarea
Carb, Merc Sol, Phosphorus, Tuberculinum. Treatment Duration - 1 to 3
months.

Oral Candiadiasis - duration 7 to 15 days associated with diarrhoea,
oesophagitis with dysphagia. Remedies - Borax, Hydrastis, Merc Sol.
Treatment duration: 10 days to 1 month.

Genital Ulcers/Warts – ulcers range from 2 days to 1 month. Warts from 3 months to 1 year. Warts could be cauliflower type and multiple. Remedies found effective – Baryta Carb, Calc Flour, Kali Bichromicum, Medorrhinum, Nux Vomica, Natrum Sulph, Nitric Acid, Phosphorus, Silicea, Staphysagria, Syphillinum, Thuja, Cantharis, Cannabis Sativa, Lycopodium, Natrum Mur. Treatment duration - 7 days to 1 month.

Herpes Zoster - from 4 days to 7 days and with fever. On chest, arms and thighs. Remedies Rhus tox, Hepar sulph. Treatment duration 10 days to 1 month.

Parotitis - a four year child suffered for 3 years. Mother of child was HIV+ with history of tuberculosis. Child was treated with Calc Iodum. Took 3 months.

Chicken Pox - This was observed in a 10-year old Thalassemic girl. Recovery with Calcarea Carb took about 10 days.

Pleural Effusion - ranging from 15 days to 1 month. Massive involvement on right. Associated with vomiting. Remedies - Arsenic Alb and Kali Carb. Treatment duration -1 to 2 months in Hospital situation. 10 days at home.

Effectiveness of Homoeopathic Treatment, Statistically Speaking

Clinical Condition	No of Cases Observed / Recovered		Effectiveness in %
Diarrhea	24	19	79
Fevers	17	12	70
Chronic Cough	25	19	76
Pruritic Dermatitis	21	21	100
Apthous Stomatitis	11	11	100
Lymphadenopathy	14	10	71
Oral Candidiasis	04	04	100
Genital ulcers/warts	27	27	100
Herpes Zoster	04	04	100
Chicken Pox	04	04	100
Pleural Effusion	02	02	100
Bilateral Parotitis	01	01	100

The body throws out toxins all the time. Strong toxins appear as rash on the skin and cause an itch. Hahnemann termed this disease-state Psora. Allopaths, without understanding the bodily processes, term them as 'skin disorders' and suppress them by ointments and antibiotics. Depending upon what was suppressed, gonorrhoea or syphillis, Hahneman termed the disease states Sycosis and Syphillis. Syphillis destroys the intellect; whereas Sycosis renders man incapable of discrimination and sane judgment, thus forming the basis of a sadistic personality. The fourth stage, Tuberculosis, is the combined effect of Psora, Sycosis and Syphillis. We are seeing the three disease states reigning supreme and combining with Vaccinosis to become AIDS and Cancers. This well considered opinion, read with explanations given through out the book, will make you realise that AIDS is a chronic condition.

Now let us look at the Allopathic Immunization: In diseases caused by the so-called viruses, in fact, homeopathy is the only system which has effectively cured, be it Small Pox or Japanese encephalitis. If, at all, modern medicine has succeeded in a limited way, in treating viral diseases with vaccines, it is by imitating homeopathy in a crude way in the method of preparation of these vaccines as well as the crude application of the principle of symptom-similarity. A case in point is that of the Poliomyelitis vaccines. Of the two kinds available, the Salk Vaccine (produced from inactivated polio virus) and the Sabin vaccine (an attenuation), the latter is more effective and has come to be accepted by the profession the world over. Like in other diseases, homeopathy has clearly established its superiority in treating viral diseases. These vaccines (called nosodes in homoeo parlance) are produced from the diseased products themselves.

Allopathic immunisation procedure itself is a health hazard. Vaccines wiped out small-pox, polio, diphtheria, typhoid, influenza, we are told. In effect, however, the blood contamination from the vaccines not only causes the same disease in severe and even fatal forms, but the vaccine poisons cause other diseases, such as, paralysis, blindness, brain damage, cancers, etc. Hence, go in for safer, cheaper, more reliable Homeopathic Prophylactics.

HERE IS A LIST OF HOMEOPATHIC VACCINES:
AIDS : Medorrhinum, Syphilinum, Tuberculinum or Thuja.
(Also, Echinacea, Lachesis, Sulphur, Phosphorus and Lycopodium).

Cancer : Carcinocin.
Chicken Pox : Malandrinum or Variolinum.
Diphtheria : Diphtherinum or Mercurious Cyanatus.
Gonorrhoea : Medorrhinum.
Infective Hepatitis : Nux Vomica.
Influenza : Arsenic Album.
Measles (Rubella) Morbillinum or Pulsatilla.
Mumps : Morbillinum or Parotidinum.
Polio : Lathyrus or polio nosode.
Rabies : Hydrophobinum (Lyssin).
Syphilis : Syphilinum.
Small Pox : Variolinum.
Tuberculosis : Bacillinum or Tuberculinum.
Typhoid : Ars Alb. or Baptisia.
Whooping Cough : Drosera or Pertusin.

For the after effects of Allopathic Vaccination or Vaccinosis, or to neutralize lethal drugs like AZT - which inhibit bone-marrow production, which in turn necessitates continual blood transfusion for many patients - give Thuja and Kali Mur and lots of fresh curds (see Diet chapter for details on curds).

And before I close this key chapter, a little bit of self help. If you or your partner is suddenly found labeled as HIV positive, you might benefit from learning about the Bach Remedies in some depth, to support you through the crisis. **They include:** *Mimulus* for fear of getting ill; *Mimulus* and *Aspen* for apprehensiveness and fear of death; *Holly* and *Willow* for anger, resentment and desire for revenge; *Gorse* for feelings of hopelessness; *Sweet chestnut* for extreme despair; *Walnut* to assist the transition in lifestyle and values; *Pine* for guilt and self-blame; *Wild rose* for apathy, resignation or collapse; *Honeysuckle* for regrets over the past.

DIET & NUTRITION IN AIDS

Food = Health. Once this fundamental truth is understood, the rest is easy to follow. If the food we eat lacks vitality, then the person ingesting that food will be operating from that lower, less energized level. Chinese call this *Chi,* Japanese call it *Qi* and Indians call it *Ojas shakti or Prana shakti.* It is an invisible life-giving nourishment that flows from the environment (internal and external) into the body. It is sometimes difficult to control our external environment but we have complete control over our internal environment - the food we eat.

It is time we became aware of the shocking reality that 90 per cent of all diseases are nutritional disorders. Ayurveda believes that food nourishes body, mind and consciousness. A proper diet, therefore, can help in gaining or maintaining weight, reducing stress and cholesterol, maintaining correct level of sugar, blood pressure, enhancing vigour, stamina, strength, vitality and mental wellbeing. Proper food is equal to proper health. Correct diet, exercise, stress reduction, a proper environment, and a healthy mental outlook all play significant roles in keeping the immune system working adequately.

Hippocrates said long ago: Let your food be your medicine. Human nutrition is the most important problem of life. We have sixteen elements in human body, which have specific tasks to perform. These elements are : Oxygen, Nitrogen, Hydrogen, Carbon, Chlorine, Flourine, Phosphorous, Iron, Calcium, Potassium, Mangnesium, Sodium, Manganese, Sulphur, Silicon and Iodine. A diet that fails to contain a certain amount of these organic salts is certainly a worthless one; for example bread, meat, potatoes and other cooked foods. This dead diet is acid forming being deprived of its alkaline requirements. It cannot harmonize the acids of the stomach. Meat, for instance, decays in the intestine. It forms gases, which get into the alimentary walls. Blood is then surcharged with waste material, which blocks the capillaries. **Chronic diseases, weakness and low vitality are traced to accumulation of waste material.**

Nutritional deficiencies can lead to immune deficiency. Zinc deficiency, in particular, leads to immunity disturbances. Studies have revealed that Vitamin A, B$_{12}$, Iron, Zinc, Folic Acid and Vitamin C can boost the immune mechanism of HIV compromised person. Consequently, in HIV/AIDS, nutrition plays an important role and diet is usually changed with emphasis on raw foods for purposes of detoxification of the lymph system and the gastro-intestinal tract. Raw vegetable juices, and the use of buttermilk or warm water enemas, may be included for detoxification. If thrush is present, mushrooms, sugar and yeast should be avoided.

People who are affected with AIDS may need a diet that helps them (a) to increase their appetite and take in enough nutrients; (b) to invigorate the digestive system to cope with and recover from diarrhoea and (c) to gain weight and strength lost during illness. Diarrhoea damages the gut, so fewer nutrients are absorbed. Damaged intestines need easily digestible foods. Fatty or oily foods can worsen diarrhoea. Milk can also cause poor absorption and intolerance in some persons due to the presence of lactose sugar found in milk. Milk can also pass on animal diseases through an already weakened immune system.

Raw salads are among the protective foods and must form a part of every meal. They not only contribute essential vitamins, minerals, amino acids, antioxidants, enzymes and phytochemicals to the diet, they also add the bulk required for proper body functions, maintaining the alkaline condition and reserves in the body. They add variety, colour, flavour and texture to diet. **Raw salads are sunlight dishes as the electro-magnetic energy of sunlight is stored in the vegetables.**

A glassful of carrot juice mixed with a desert spoonful of fresh amla juice and a tablespoonful of honey taken once or twice daily, for example, is a very effective natural tonic. It increases body resistance against colds and infections, improves complexion and weight, prevents amnesia, hair loss, debilitating weakness and adverse effects of chemotherapy, night blindness, early aging and protects nerves, brain, heart, lungs and liver. Carotenoids (in yellow vegetables) and lycopene (found in tomatoes) helps the body in thwarting the Cancer-causing process known as oxidation. Once on a diet of raw plant-food the body can cleanse and heal itself, sending energy levels soaring.

Johanna Brandt, the author of 'The Grape Cure' advocates an exclusive grape diet to cleanse the body of the dead cells/cancers. After a 'water-only' fast of two to three days, she puts her patients on an exclusive grape diet. The patient takes a grape meal every two hours from 8 am to 8 pm. One begins with 30, 60 to 90 grams per meal. The treatment may last anywhere from two weeks to three months, depending upon the severity of illness and the type of constitution, mental make-up of a patient, environmental factors, etc.

Dr. Ann Wigmore of 'Be Your Own Doctor' fame, likewise, propounds **Wheat Grass Therapy** for about 300 diseases. The active ingredient of Wheat Grass is Chlorophyll, which contains almost all the mineral and vitamins. Fresh juice of wheat grass contains Vitamins A, B, B_{17}, C and K, and also carbohydrates, proteins, etc. Scientists like Dr. Burser call it the concentrated solar energy. Others call it the nectar of life. Dr. Ann Wigmore calls it the Green Blood.

The contents of Chlorophyll in Wheat Grass and of Hemin in Hemoglobin of Blood are 99% similar. The arrangement of molecular structure of Carbon, Hydrogen, Oxygen and Nitrogen are very much similar in Chlorophyll and Hemin, except a little change in the centre. Magnesium is the centre of Chlorophyll molecule, while we find Iron in the Centre of Hemin Molecule.

AIDS victims must have alkaline diet, naturally grown food with high vitamin and mineral content and low in proteins. In fact animal proteins, which are touted as very effective body-builders, are the main cause of cancers and other viral load. If the body is strong, AIDS or any other virus will not attack, as food builds up the regenerative forces of the body. AIDS and Cancer patients must have ONLY raw diet consisting of fruits, vegetables, salads, fruit juices for about three months to detoxify their bodies. Yellow bananas, papaya and also jack fruit are excellent foods for AIDS patients. French scientists found that the extract of jackfruit, called jacaline, inhibited the growth of the AIDS-causing human immune deficiency virus in test tubes during experiments. The power of jacaline was discovered by Jean Favero from the microbiology and immunology section of the French National Institute of Health and Medical Research (INSERM) in 1993.

Therefore, HIV/AIDS patients should increase their intake of fresh fruits and vegetables, organically grown if possible (avoiding foods that have been treated with pesticides and other sprays), plus lentils, beans, seeds, nuts and whole grains, including brown rice and millet. Raw foods are particularly important because cooking depletes foods of their vital enzymes. Cruciferous vegetables, such as, broccoli, Brussels sprouts, cabbage, and cauliflower and yellow and deep-orange vegetables, such as, carrots, pumpkin, squash, and yams should be taken in plenty by PLWAs.

They should also eat semi ripened papaya, yellow bananas, fresh pineapple frequently. These foods are good sources of proteolytic enzymes, which are crucial for proper digestion of foods and assimilation of nutrients. Without enzymes, the body cannot be supplied with the energy. It is also necessary to eliminate from the diet colas, foods with additives and colorings, junk foods, peanuts, processed refined foods, saturated fats, salt, sugar and sugar products, white flour, all animal protein, and anything that contains caffeine.

AIDS patients should also exercise caution in their choice of foods so as to avoid exposure to food-borne illness. Food poisoning can be very dangerous for people with AIDS. They should not smoke, and must stay away from those who do. Also, avoid alcohol, noxious chemicals, and everything else that can damage the liver. Determine what food sensitivities or allergies may be present. It is important to eliminate allergenic foods from the diet because they wreak havoc in the body, causing damage to the immune system.

"You are as young as your glands; you are as young as your cells; you are as young as your collagen; you are as young as your digestive and assimilative system; you are as young as your arteries; you are as young as your mind", writes Dr. Paavo Airola in his famous book Rejuvenation Secrets. He adds : "But in order to keep your glands and organs young and efficient, your digestive tract free from decay and putrefaction, your cells well oxygenated, healthy and vital, your collagen elastic, your arteries open and free from cholesterol, and your mind clear and efficient, you have to feed your body with the highest quality nutrition – nutrition which will supply your glands, organs, and tissues with all the nutrients essential for normal, healthy, and efficient functioning. So, you can see that the ultimate secret of staying young is basically the secret of staying healthy. And, the secret of staying healthy is closely tied to proper nutrition".

In other words, if we have to maintain health, vigour and vitality, our blood stream should be 70% alkaline and 30% acidic. But because of the wrong kind of food that we ingest, this ratio is usually in inverse proportion. This faulty blood keeps on circulating affecting the organs like brain, heart, lungs, kidneys, etc. As a result, vital force diminishes and one gets diseased.

It is, therefore, necessary to note the difference between 'alkaline/laxative foods' and 'acidic/constipating foods'. It is well to remember that pickles, ketchup, mustard, pepper, vinegar, spices, etc. have no nutritive value and are harmful to the body. Salt should be used sparingly. Tea and coffee are harmful. Cocoa and chocolate should be used sparingly. White bread, pork, cheese, baked beans, corned beef, fat meats, rich puddings, dumplings, pies, cakes, sausages and all fried foods are difficult to digest. Sweet milk should not be used at the same meal with meat.

Remember these are laxative foods : Apples, plums, peaches, oranges, pears, grapefruit, pineapples, grapes, figs, prunes, spinach, cauliflower, tomatoes, lettuce, onions, turnips, celery, parsnips, oatmeal, raisins, green peas, cabbage (raw), carrots, string beans, dandelion greens, beet-top greens, buttermilk, whole wheat, bran.

And these are constipating foods : White bread, pastry, cornstarch, sago, sweet milk, cheese, eggs, rice, tea, coffee, salt meat, pickled meat, mixed dishes, spiced foods, white crackers.

Perfect Food : The perfect food consists of honey, hot water, oat-meal, lemon juice, grated apples and ground hazel-nuts which contain all the vitamins. Soak ten almonds in water at night. Remove the skin and take them in the morning with one or two tablespoonfuls of honey. This is a potent brain tonic. Try to live on butter- milk and/or fruits once a week at least.

Vitamins A, C and E are also very important, but in natural form, if you want to stay away from cancer. Citrus fruits, dark green and deep yellow vegetables, cabbage, broccoli and cauliflower contain a chemical that can inhibit HIV/AIDS. **Dr. Fukunir Morishige** (noted Japanese scientist) after 30 years of painstaking research has found that Vitamin C and copper compound has lethal effects on cancer. This very principle can be used in AIDS cure.

Orange juice mixed with fresh grape juice makes a good tonic. This is ideal in anaemia, general debility, rickets, etc. Plantain contains A, B, C and D vitamins plus phosphorous and iron. It is a very nutritious fruit. It promotes growth, augments vigour and adds flesh to the body. A fully ripe banana is laxative. Mangoes contain sugar and highly refined turpentine in them. They also contain iron and other useful acids. They are useful in rheumatism, diarrhoea, diabetes, etc. Pomegranates are also very invigorating, cooling and strengthening. The juice is refreshing and toning and soothes sore throats.

Therefore, consume plenty of fresh juices. They help in throwing out toxins, diseased cells and dead matter from the blood and other organs. Green drinks made from leafy greens, such as, kale, spinach, and beet greens, and carrot and beet root juice, should be consumed on a daily basis, with garlic and onion added. This is a great tonic for anaemia, and of utmost benefit in thalassemia and leukemia.

Another very effective method to detoxify your body is to drink lots of water and eat raw, natural, organic foods, which have high water content. For instance, consuming mainly raw vegetable juice (about 500 ml) is a classic detox technique. Vegetables with good detox potential are carrots, cucumber, pumpkin, spinach, beetroot and tomato. Eat about one kilo of fruits like fresh apricots, citrus fruits, papaya, peaches, melons and all types of berries, for three consecutive days every alternate month.

Read all about Fruit Juice Coctails in AIDS and other diseases, on the following page .....

FRUIT JUICES

Many common ailments respond favourably when raw juices are taken. Some disorders and the juices most beneficial to them are listed below :

AIDS : jackfruit, yellow bananas, papaya, black grapes, carrot, spinach, grapefruit, lemon and radish.

Allergies : apricot, grapes, carrot, parsley.

Anaemia : apricot, prune, strawberry, beetroot, parsley, spinach, carrot.

Arthritis : apple, cherry, lemon, grapefruit, cucumber, beetroot, carrot, celery, watercress.

Bladder ailments : apple, apricot, lemon, cucumber, carrot, celery, parsley, watercress.

Colds : orange, lemon, grapefruit, pineapple, carrot, onion.

Coughs (including bronchitis and asthma) : grapes, orange, lemon, carrot, radish, celery.

Constipation : apricot, orange, pear, plum, prune, carrot, beetroot, spinach, watercress.

Diarrhoea : apple, carrot, celery.

Dental problems : apple, grapes, tomato, carrot, spinach.

Eye troubles : apricot, tomato, carrot, celery, parsley, spinach, papaya.

Halitosis : apple, grapefruit, lemon, pineapple, tomato, carrot, celery, spinach.

Gall stones : apricot, lemon, grapefruit, tomato, beetroot, carrot, parsley.

Headaches : grape, lemon, tomato, lettuce, parsley, cucumber, beet.

High BP : orange, lemon, pear, pineapple, cucumber, parsley, beetroot.

Influenza : apple, grape, lemon, lettuce, carrot, celery.

Kidney trouble : orange, lemon, carrot, celery, watercress, beetroot, parsley, cucumber, apple.

Low BP : grapes, apricot, carrot.

Migraine : grapes, lemon, tomato, lettuce, parsley, spinach.

Overweight : grapes, lemon, pear, plum, peach, pineapple, strawberry, cabbage, lettuce, spinach, carrot.

Rheumatism : cherry, grapes, orange, grapefruit, strawberry, cucumber, beetroot, carrot, watercress.

Tonsillitis : apricot, lemon, orange, grapefruit, pineapple, prune, carrot, spinach, radish.

Varicose veins : grape, orange, plum, tomato, beetroot, carrot, spinach, radish.

AIDS and Cancer patients will especially benefit from Dr. Gerson program, which is described below, because these chronic diseases are the result of accumulated toxins and deficiencies in the body over the years.

When juice is drunk, it enters the blood stream almost as fast as alcohol, providing all the required nutrients to the body. Dr. Gerson, who pioneered this treatment, required his patients to drink one 8 ounce glass of juice 13 times a day.

Drinking such large quantities of fresh juice everyday dislodges accumulated body poisons, which are absorbed by the liver, somewhat overburdening it. To help out the liver, the Gerson approach employs an unusual detoxification technique. Organic, body-temperature coffee is administered rectally which stimulates the bile ducts of the liver to dump scavenged toxins into the colon for evacuation. Coffee enema also helps in reviwing a person in coma.

How coffee enema is prepared: Boil 1 quart distilled water, add 3 tablespoons drip ground coffee, reduce heat, and simmer for 15 minutes. Strain and add sufficient water to again have 1 quart. Cool to body temperature, and then introduce eight inches into the colon with an enema kit. Retain the enema for 12 to 15 minutes.

"Salt is the worst poison taken in excess", averred Dr.Gerson and added that it caused displacement of potassium found naturally in human cells, leaving them vulnerable to attack by disease. Therefore, he put his patients on very-low-sodium, but potassium-rich diet. Supplemental potassium in the form of equal parts of potassium gluconate, potassium acetate, and mono potassium phosphate was given to balance the sick body. Flaxseed oil was the preferred fatty acid source, and was to be 'raw and cold' and not to be used for cooking. Pancreatin, acidophilus, and vitamin B_3 (niacin) were also provided supplementally.

The most common criticisms of the Gerson program are that the diet is restrictive and that the coffee enemas are excessive. It is true that the Gerson therapy is an extreme diet, but then AIDS and cancers can be desribed as extreme conditions. One extreme may call for another; it takes a lot of water to put out a burning building. If the 'all knowing' (read not knowing anything) oncologists can use deadly chemical, radiological and surgical extremes, why not extreme nutrition? At least it will not do harm like the carcinogens pumped into frail bodies of AIDS and cancer patients.

Finally, we have the best panacea for AIDS. Its name is **curds** (yogurts, thyre, *dahi*). It has been used for zillions of years as the most effective, safest, cheapest, very readily available 'medicine' all over the world. Much before an India-born Dr. Bharat Ramratnam, an HIV specialist at Brown Medical School, Rhode Island, and his colleagues changed the genetic make-up of the bacteria *Lactococcus Lactis* so that it generated *Cyanovirin*, a drug that has prevented HIV infection in monkeys and human cells (The Times of India, 19 January 2006), the prostitutes all over the world have been using fresh curds mixed with turmeric and sour lime as a preventive for all kinds of STDs, vaginal ulcers, etc.

Let it be firmly ingrained in your mind that improper diet causes diseases and consequently proper diet alone can cure all those diseases. Right diet and lifestyle compliment the body's wondrous mechanism for growth, stamina, repair and physical as well as mental well-being. The only cocktail that I drink and prescribe is the fruit juice cocktail. (Lest you misunderstand, I am not HIV positive. But I am positive that HIV does not cause AIDS).

In short, Diet is the best Doctor. The other most wonderful doctors of the world are: Dr. Air, Dr. Pure Water, Dr. Sleep, Dr. Sunshine, Dr. Exercises, Dr. Smile, Dr. Love, Dr. Care and Dr. Leo Rebello. If you were to follow the advice of these ten doctors properly, you will live to be healthy hundred without ills, pills and doctor's bills.

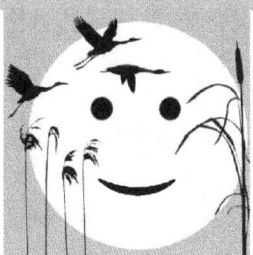

BIO-TESTING & BIO-THERAPY
A MEDICAL BREAKTHROUGH IN ARRESTING
THE SPREAD OF AIDS & CANCER

In every country, people are being vaccinated. X-rays taken in hospitals leave behind poisonous residue in the body, medicines regularly taken also leave behind toxic matter. Dental amalgams (like mercury and silver) too lead to metal poisoning. All these settle in the body tissues. These poisons block blood circulation in the fine capillaries and impede the secretion of lymphatic glands. The build-up of these toxins in the body leads to the gradual deterioration of health. Many kinds of diseases ranging from pituitary gland intoxication, heart, liver, pancreas poisoning occur, leading to arthritis, asthma, weak immunity, etc.

If there exists a method for removing malaria parasites from the blood and cleansing the brain of meningococcus virus in a matter of minutes, it must be recognised as a medical breakthrough. This is precisely what can be achieved with Bio-testing and Bio-therapy. This unique scientific system, pioneered by the German doctor R.Voll and perfected by Rev. Dr. Fred Fox using Radionics (vibrations) and tapes, is being used in UK and India.

This therapy is based on the precise matching of the needs of the patient's life force with energies radiated by homeopathic remedies. These remedies radiate energies of various plants, minerals etc. from which they are derived. When the energy of the remedy matches up with the energy radiated by a particular organ or function of the body, it can be used to tune and detoxify the body.

A unique method is used to diagnose a patient. Dr. Voll discovered that by touching the adductor muscle, which exists in the web of one's hand from the thumb to the forefinger, 'bio points' of the body can be easily and objectively tested. If the adductor muscle goes into a spasm, the practitioner knows that there is some toxicity in the vascular system related to the bio points. The muscle reaction in the webbing of the hand relates to a reaction of the thymus. It shares sympathetic innervations through the second thoracic ganglia on the spine. Since the thymus is central immune tissue, the reaction in the muscle indicates an immune system reaction. Hence, it's great diagnostic value.

To treat the patient, a combination of remedies, which are recorded on magnetic tapes in glass vials, are placed in the patient's palm. Dr. Fox discovered that remedies could be applied simply and effectively by placing them in the patient's palm and then lightly tapping on the patient's arm, shoulder or thighs. Each tap stimulates the life force sufficiently to expel toxins from the areas of the body. This is regarded as 'Applied Homeopathy' and is different from the conventional remedy of pills.

Thus, this method is an invaluable latest methodology to:
1.. Diagnose the cause of the toxicity build-up in the body.
2.. Identify the poisons trapped in the body tissues.
3.. Locate the body areas where the toxic matter is concentrated.
4.. Remove the toxic matter by helping the body to manufacture anti-toxins using radionics vibrationary methods combating microbial/chemical toxicity by biochemic tissue salts, homeopathic and flower remedies, magnets, colour therapy and acupressure.

As the therapy works for removal of bacteria and viruses and clearing of chemicals and toxins from the body and aura of the patient, this therapy has produced very encouraging results for cases of HIV/AIDS, Cancers, tuberculosis, meningitis, hepatitis, malaria, heart and kidney complications etc. The treatment, which takes about an hour to an hour-and-a-half, is a complete treatment in itself and does not require sophisticated gadgets, hospitalisation, surgery or costly medicines.

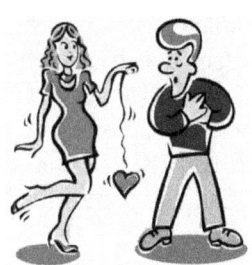

OXYGEN SHORTAGE DISEASES

One has only to hold one's breath for a few seconds to understand how dependent we are on oxygen support. A mere four minutes without oxygen can cause permanent damage to the human brain. Ten minutes without can cause death. Adequately oxygenated, the body is strong, energetic and disease-free; the mind is clear and sharp. Without adequate oxygen, various unpleasant symptoms can occur, like fatigue, foggy mind and headaches to debilitating and life-threatening illnesses - all of which are often mistakenly attributed to other factors. There is growing evidence that the increasing rate of cancers and other diseases worldwide are directly linked to the decline in available oxygen. In medical jargon they are called hypoxic diseases.

DID YOU KNOW... *That* atmospheric oxygen is declining. *That* over many cities levels may fall as low as 12% from earlier levels of around 30%? *That* a healthy human body is made up of around 4/5 water, and that water is 8/9 oxygen? *That* the darker the blood color, the less oxygen it carries? *That* antibiotics kill friendly bacteria which produce H_2O_2 (hydrogen peroxide) and, consequently, reduce oxygen in the body? *That* phytoplankton and rain forests each normally recycle 50% of the Earth's oxygen? *That* phytoplankton growth can be multiplied 50 times faster by designed fertilization? *That* oxygen therapy is being successfully used to treat ailments, from cancer and multiple sclerosis to AIDS, arthritis and Alzheimer's disease?

Factors that deplete Oxygen in the human body are : Reduction of oxygen in the atmosphere; burning fossil fuels; polluted/fluoridated water; consumption of heavy meat diets and highly processed foods; medicines toxic to healthy cells; tobacco and substance abuse; mineral deficiencies; overeating; improper breathing techniques; stress and negative mind-set; infections. **Available oxygen therapies include:** Oxygen bars/portable oxygen. Stabilized oxygen supplements and H_2O_2 supplemental beverages. Super-oxidated water. Hyperbaric oxygen treatment. Chelation therapy. But no individual therapies can make up for depleted oxygen supplies in the atmosphere for most of Earth's six billion (and more) population! **Pollute less and do regular *pranayama.***

KAI IGAKU
HOW DOES *KAI IGAKU* (WELLNESS MEDICINE) WORK?

In *Kai Igaku,* diagnosis is done by a proven method of kinesiology. This method is called the Life Energy Test. It is easy to learn and you can test a person on: **(a)** weak or strong immunity, **(b)** weak or strong organs, **(c)** viruses, bacteria, parasites and other pathological conditions, and **(d)** appropriate medicines, herbs and nutrition. The only things you need for this test are: two persons to check the patient; a copper or metal stick of a few inches; and sheets with photos or photocopies of pathological conditions.

The person can have a full diagnosis including a test of helpful medicines within one hour, something that would take a modern hospital weeks of testing. In Nicaragua they have compared their results with the clinical tests of a standard scientific medical research institute, and the rate of same results was over 80%. The one very remarkable result was that the kinesiological test was more accurate than the clinical test in finding out if someone has cancer. Initial herbal treatment of the kidneys and urine therapy in the form of a few drops (or a homeopathic dilution) would solve the problem.

THE GENERAL RECIPE FOR TREATMENT IS:
1) drinking of 2-3 litres of herbal teas, tested kinesiologically; **2)** change of diet: no meat, no sugar, no refined or chemical products, lots of vegetables and fruits instead; **3)** drinking urine: from one glass in minor ailments up to 2-3 litres a day in serious conditions; **4)** massage and mud packs with urine; **5)** hot foot-baths with water, tested herbal teas and urine; **6)** warmth treatments on the vital organs (in Japanese called *soto*); **7)** simple and pleasant physical movement-exercises (in Japanese called *sotai*).

The immune system normally reacts very fast on intensive urine therapy supported by the herbal teas and partial or total fasting. They have had many cases where, in the course of a few weeks, cancers and tumors disappeared. No hospitalization, no toxic treatments, fast results: your own medicine, your own water of life, no cost, always there! Even in the cases where people died of cancer after all, the dying process was much different. There was less or no pain, the person was calm and relatively happy and often conscious till the end. We often forget that death is not a failure and that a good death belongs to healing as well. Urine therapy makes a wonderful contribution and is on deeper level nectar of immortality.

Urine is a byproduct. It is 95% water and contains hormones, enzymes, vitamins, minerals and tissue salts. These substances can stimulate the immune system and fight infections. Dr. Shigeyuri Arai (from Japan) avers that gargling with urine alone can cure many diseases including cancer, hepatitis B, influenza and host of other diseases, ranging from common cold to diabetes. Before undertaking auto urine therapy, one needs to fast for three days and avoid flesh food, alcohol, tobacco, etc. In that case, urine tastes like coconut water and is the elixir of life.

HOMEOPATHIC URINE AND DETOXIFICATION

In many cases of modern immune disorders there is toxification of the tissues and cells by heavy metals and ethyls (petroleum-derivatives). Often one can guide these toxins out of the body by using homeopathic remedies, like *mercurius vivus* D_6, *plumbum metallicum* D_{12}, *amalgam* D_6. Some of those toxic substances have bound themselves to other substances, etc. They do not respond to homeopathic detoxification dilutions. These aggressive metabolites can be found in small quantities in the urine. When one uses this urine (in small quantity), the body is able to react and starts to detoxify these substances, stimulated on the energetic level.

HOW TO MAKE HOMEOPATHIC URINE

*Take 6 little bottles of 10 ml each and fill these with approx. 9 ml clean water.
* Take 15 drops of fresh urine and drop these into bottle no. 1.
* Hold bottle no. 1 horizontally in your right hand and hit 20 times on the other hand. Now you have a homeopathic potency D_1.
* Take 15 drops out of bottle no. 1 and put them in bottle no.2. Repeat the rest of the procedure.
* Do this till you have finished with the last bottle and then you have the potencies D_1 till D_6, ready for use.
* You can test kinesiologically which potency is best; but you can also take 5 drops from each bottle.
* You can repeat this procedure each day to have updated detoxification information.

MAGNETO-THERAPY

Magneto-therapy is the art of healing through magnets. The application of magnets relieves and cures many distressing diseases without medicine.

Coupled with diet change, internal cleansing by means of fasting, hydrotherapy and yogic kriyas, magneto-therapy works wonders.

Magneto-therapy is easy, safe, and simple, yet quick in some cases. There is no adverse effect, reaction or shock. It is economical as the same magnets can be used by hundreds of persons for various ailments for years together. If the magnets lose their power, they can be recharged to regain fresh strength.

Magneto-therapy is very beneficial in arthritis, asthma, backaches, bed-wetting, boils, bronchitis, cancer, cervical spondylosis, diseases of bowels and uterus, rheumatism, sciatica, sleeplessness, sprains, stiffness, swellings, toothache, etc.

CASE STUDIES
Arthritis : Apply North pole to affected part for 10 to 15 minutes, twice daily.
Bleeding, menstrual : sit on the North pole for 10 to 15 minutes.
Blood clots : apply North Pole over the clots till they disappear.
Blood Pressure, High : south pole of medium powered magnet under the right ear.
Bones, broken : North pole at the broken joint with South pole slightly higher above.
Brain, tumours : North pole of medium powered magnet over the skull for 15 minutes minimum, twice daily.
Bronchitis : North pole against nose, throat and lungs for 5 minutes at each location.
Cancerous growth : North pole locally for 15 minutes. Also, eat plenty of grapes.
Digestion, weak and gases : South pole of medium or high powered magnet to the stomach, about two hours after eating.

Ear, aches, swellings, etc. : North pole from 5 to 10 minutes till result is achieved.

Emotions : For over aggressiveness sit on North pole; if slow or dull, sit on the South pole. Once a day sitting for 15 minutes.

Eyes, cataracts : North pole to the affected eye 5 to 10 minutes, twice a day.

Glaucoma : North pole to the outer edge of the affected eye, 10 minutes twice daily.

Hair Colouring : Sit on the South pole for 15 to 20 minutes before going to bed at night. Maintain regularity.

Headaches, Neuralgias : south pole against the lower stomach. Good results on empty stomach.

Heart problems : Apply South pole for 5 to 10 minutes. Medium powered magnet.

Kidney disorders : North pole of high powered magnet on the back in the kidney region for 15 minutes.

Liver dysfunctions : North pole for 15 to 20 minutes. Medium or high powered magnets depending on the problem.

Muscles : north pole for weak muscles. South pole for stiff muscles, 10 minutes.

Piles : Sit on the North Pole 10 to 15 minutes twice a day. After pain has reduced use South pole. Eat laxative foods and avoid constipation.

Shoulders, Neuritis : North pole for 10 to 15 minutes.

Spine, Curved : use South pole where the curve is prominent and North pole on the opposite side.

Teeth and Gums : North pole for 15 to 20 minutes.

Throat : for infection use North pole 10 minutes. For weak throat use South pole for 5 to 10 minutes.

Thyroid, inflamed : North pole, 10 minutes each on both sides.

These are general instructions. Special cases need expert attention.

YOGA & AIDS

Yoga teachers who are interested in teaching HIV/AIDS patients should gain some basic familiarity with AIDS before venturing out to teach. An understanding of how AIDS can be transmitted is critical. Some PLWAs may have open sores or wounds, may vomit in class, or may have nosebleeds. Yoga teachers must be prepared to deal with these situations safely. In addition, basic knowledge about some of the opportunistic infections that accompany AIDS is important. For those with a red rash, itching, or redness of the eyes, one should avoid the full inversions and backbends to prevent overheating, and instead focus on supported forward bends. Just one session of forward bends can bring significant improvement to a red rash. Students with retinitis should avoid the full inversions. Those who have recently had a bout of pneumocystis pneumonia should practice the more gentle backbends and avoid exertion as it may prove dangerous to delicate lung cells.

It is dinned into you, day in and day out that the AIDS virus infects and kills helper T cells, the front-line troops of the immune system by weakening the thymus. Yoga helps rejuvenate thymus, which in turn direct T-cells to recognize the invader and mobilize killer T cells and B cell antibodies and defend the body. The AIDS virus (official name HTLV-III, or human T cell lymphotropic virus type III; also called HIV) is transmitted in several ways: (a) by direct contact of the skin or mucous membrane (as in the rectum, mouth or vagina) with infected semen, blood, and possibly also saliva; (2) by transfusion of infected blood products; and (3) by sharing of contaminated intravenous blood paraphernalia.

Yoga can halt or reverse the progression of AIDS. Scientists are discovering what folk wisdom has always known: You can worry yourself sick. You can grieve yourself to death. Out of this research has emerged a new branch in medicine called : **psychoneuroimmunology,** a blend of psychology, neurology and immunology. And to those who are open, it brings insights into the long-known salutary effects of yoga on health. *Good nutrition, proper exercise, adequate sleep, relaxation, meditation,* *breathing practice of paced respiration, enhances the immune function. Whereas, poor diet, inactivity, insomnia, somnolence, constant stress, smoking, heavy alcohol consumption, depresses the immune function.*

Yoga is not a religion. It is a way of life. It is an eight-fold path of evolution from a man to a superman. Yoga gives preference to health rather than to strength. Yoga secures perfect health, with complete biological and mental control. With regular Yoga, we can have sound health, sound mind, meaningful existence, peace, happiness and self-realization. Yoga considers prevention of disease very vital. Yoga teaches you to relax and live your life to the full.

WHAT YOGA CAN DO FOR YOU ?

a) *Sharp Alert Mind* with increased power of concentration, of efficiency and precision. **b)** *Ability to Relax*, to invigorate yourself mentally and physically, if you are tired. **c)** *Emotional Control* resulting in poise, fortitude and equanimity by elimination of all problems, tensions which lead to stress condition. **d)** *Mental Harmony and Peace* within oneself, and a meaningful life.

In yoga we have exercises for most chronic diseases, such as, tuberculosis, asthma, bronchitis, liver disorders, hypertension, diabetes, spinal defects, arthritis, rheumatism, eye defects, psychological disorders, leprosy, renal failure, heart cases and a host of other diseases. In fact, in Yoga we do not compartmentalize anything. The body is a unit and it works as a whole. Treat the whole body and you are fine.

Let us now look at some Asanas to illustrate the point. *Suryanamaskar* (12 variations of Sun-bathing and limbering) and *Sarvangasana* (shoulder stand) are specific in the treatment of leprosy, coupled with foods rich in sulphur (like raw cabbage and cauliflower) and fresh, cow-milk to tone up the endocrine system. *Paschimtanasan* (posterior stretching), *Ardha-Matsyendrasana* (lateral twist) and *Dhanurasana* (bow pose) are the postures used in the cure of Diabetes and cleansing techniques. You need not take insulin injection for life.

Paschimtanasan is also used for epilepsy and gastro-intestinal disorders with good results along with fasting. *Bhujangasana* (cobra pose), *Shalabhasana* (locust posture) and *Matsyasana* (fish pose) are performed for the cure of asthma, bronchitis and tuberculosis, among other disorders.

Viparit-Karani (elbow stand), *Sarvangasana* (shoulder stand), *Shirshasana* (head stand), for example, are beneficial in hernia, amnesia, seminal weakness, piles, varicose veins, menstrual disorders, cerebral anaemia, prolapse of the uterus and congestion. *Makarasana* (crocodile pose), *Long Swing* and *Shavasana* (corpse pose) are used for insomnia, hypertension, heart ailments and psychological disturbances. *Tolangulasana* corrects obesity and expands chest and removes low backache.

Then you have *Tadasana* (upward stretch) for height gain, *Chakrasana* (standing lateral bending) to regularise bowel movements, *Nauli Kriya* (abdominal recti gyration) to remove constipation and cure dyspepsia, colitis, etc. Also, the Eye exercises for myopia, hypermetropia, cataract, squint, glaucoma, trachoma, diplopia; the Neck exercises for cervical spondylosis, stiff neck, frozen shoulder; and the Lumber gyration for seminal congestion, low backache, and other Yoga techniques that will give you a sure cure.

Dr. Robin Monro of the United Kingdom, some years ago conducted a Yoga Therapy Survey. Following are some of the excellent results revealed by the said survey.

Yoga Therapy Effectiveness in Percentage	% Helped
a) Back Disorders	94%
b) Asthma/Bronchitis	75%
c) Hypertension	33%
d) Heart disorders	50%
e) Duodenal ulcers	67%
f) Haemorrhoids	60%
g) Diseases of nervous or muscular systems (e.g. multiple sclerosis, Parkinsonism)	86%
h) Cancers	71%

i) Diabetes	85%
j) Rheumatism or Arthritis	83%
k) Pre-menstrual tension	82%
l) Other menstrual disorders	69%
m) Menopause disorders	83%
n) Obesity	62%
o) Migraine	65%
p) Insomnia	70%
q) Excessive anxiety	95%
r) Heavy smoking	71%
s) Alcoholism	83%

A study of Yoga, conducted in September - December 1998, by the SNDT Women's University in Bombay, confirms that Yoga can build bodily resistance and increase immunity level. The study was conducted in the Albless Hospice, which is the only residential home for HIV positive persons in Bombay. Yoga was implemented through a step-by-step procedure for four months. The candidates practiced the exercises twice a week, for an hour and half. In addition to the asanas, the candidates also practiced relaxation, pranayam and dhyana. It was seen that seven persons showed an increase in weight. Regular practice of yoga made the subjects more active and energetic. Their blood pressure showed drastic improvement. Anxiety and depression vanished making them calm, which in turn helped them to sleep well and recoup. The yogic exercises also helped reduce physical ailments, such as, back pain, digestive disturbances and improved the blood circulation. The respondents felt more at peace with self.

Yoga is beneficial for digestive complaints due to its ability to activate the parasympathetic nervous system to nourish and activate digestion and elimination. Yoga also has a regulating effect on the enteric nervous system, which independently functions, to digest, move and eliminate our food. Yoga can also be used to balance the digestive fire or *Agni*. If *Agni* is low then digestion becomes weak creating symptoms of diarrhea, bloating, gas. If *Agni* is excessive then there is much heat in the GI system creating symptoms of constipation, acid reflux, and burning. Constipation alternating with Diarrhoea, as we know, is the major problem of AIDS patients. Therefore, depending on the condition of the AIDS patient, energizing standing yoga postures and *Kapalabhati* and *Ujjayi pranayams* (to stimulate *Agni*) or supine postures and *Sitcari* and *Shitali pranayams* (to stimulate *Agni*) may be prescribed.

Yoga, likewise, helps in AIDS dementia (forgetfulness), depression, in overcoming suicidal thoughts, fears or insecurity, in lack of concentration, psychological trauma, mental imbalance, acidity, ulcers, burning caused by anti-retroviral drugs, etc.

Advantages of Yoga Techniques
a) Increase tone of voluntary and involuntary muscles and improve functional capacity of ligaments, tendons and small internal muscles.
b) Besides physical endurance, help to increase stress competence.
c) Control obesity.
d) Increase resistance to disease.
e) Heart gets massage due to the actions of the diaphragm, thereby improving the tone and function of the myocardium.
f) Brings soothing effects on both body and mind.
g) Improves respiratory function and autonomic balance.
h) Ischaemic ECG changes and decreases.
i) Due to their influence on brain and glands, the neuro-muscular coordination improves, which in turn helps develop varied skills.
j) Quickens the return of venous blood. Improves glucose tolerance.
k) Reduces cholesterol. Helps to increase longevity without exertion.

NOW LET US LOOK AT THE THERAPEUTIC BENEFITS OF A FEW ASANAS

Padmasana : improves memory, concentration and digestion. Corrects ailments of heart and mind. Strengthens lungs, expands chest. Makes the spine supple and strong.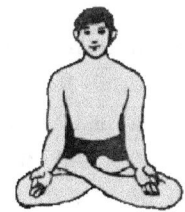

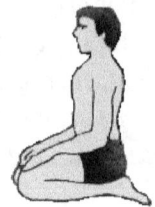

Vajrasana and Supta Vajrasana : Vajrasana is the only asana which can be performed on a full belly. It improves digestion, helps in dyspepsia, constipation, colitis, seminal weakness and eases the stiffness of the legs. Corrects ailments of thighs, calves, abdomen, spinal column and lumbar region.

Yoga Mudra : helps in proper development of hands, legs, lumbar and back. Strengthens chest and lungs. Helps in tonsillitis and asthma. Activates *Kundalini.*

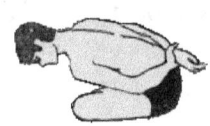

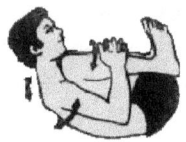

Pawana Muktasana : helps in easing constipation and gases. Removes displacements, defects of the spine. Improves the spread of back and shoulders.

Dhanurasana : corrects ailments of spinal column, neck, hands, legs, abdomen and chest. Gastro-intestinal ailments, dysentery are removed. Improves digestion and corrects obesity.

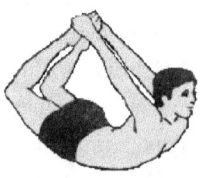

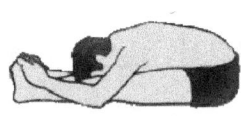

Paschimtanasan : specific for epilepsy also corrects piles and diabetes. Improves the spinal column, leg muscles and stomach tone. Waistline is trimmed. Regular practice of this posture helps in gaining height.

Sarvangasana : keeps the thyroid, thymus healthy. Beneficially influences the pelvic organs. Useful in curing varicose veins, piles, hernias, menstrual disorders. Persons with cervical spondylosis should not do this asana.

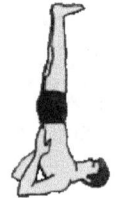

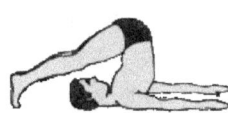

Halasan : Good for the neck, spine, liver and endocrine glands. Corrects acidity, diabetes, hydrocele and hernia. Also removes flatulence.

Tolangulasana : corrects kidney ailments, obesity. Good for strengthening hand and leg muscles and expansion of chest. Specific for reducing big botties.

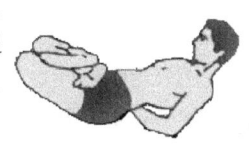

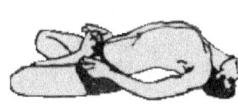

Matsyasana : corrects asthma, bronchitis and other lung disorders. Also good for diabetes, constipation and acidity. In this asana one can float in water like a fish.

Garudasana : corrects inguinal, scrotal, uterine and vaginal hernias. Also good for curing hydrocele and strengthening the leg muscles.

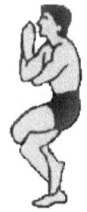

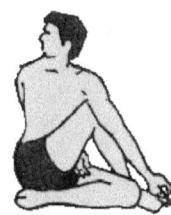

Ardha-Matsyendrasan : builds a healthy and elastic spinal column. Removes abdominal congestion. Enlarged liver, congested spleen, sluggish and inactive kidneys are improved. Specific in Diabetes, helps in constipation and dyspepsia.

Shalabhasan : lessens problems of the womb, menstruation and vaginal discharge. Low back, leg pains are eliminated. Laziness is washed out. Virility improves.

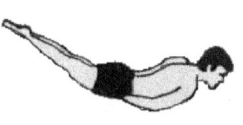

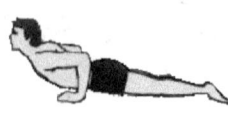

Bhujangasana : useful in cervical spondylosis, kyphosis, asthma, bronchitis and backaches. Kidneys, liver and the pancreas are also toned up. Corrects ailments of hands, semen, spinal column.

Mayurasana : this asana keeps the old age at bay. Digestive organs are toned up due to pressure exerted on the viscera. Digestive complaints vanish. It injects new energy.

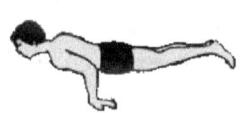

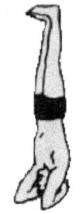

Shirshasana : functions of the brain are improved. Sense organs become efficient. The pituitary, the thyroid and the parathyroid get a rich supply of blood and excretions get regulated. It influences the nervous system and the endocrine glands. Useful in curing neurasthenia, dyspepsia, congested throat, liver and spleen, hernias, seminal weakness and asthma of the nervous and hepatic types. It also gives better eyesight.

Makarasana : good for insomnia, high blood pressure, nervousness and indigestion.

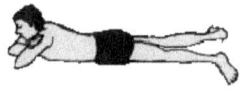

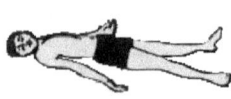

Shavasana : good for heart ailments, high blood pressure patients. Mental disorders, those having suicidal or criminal tendencies improve. Excellent for relaxation.

YOGA PRACTICES BENEFICIAL FOR HIV-AIDS PATIENTS ARE : *Padmasana* (the lotus pose ideal for meditation), *Sarvangasan* (shoulder stand), *Yoga Mudra in Vajrasan* (child pose), *Bhujangasana* (cobra pose), *Matsyasana* (fish pose), *Shalabhasan* (the locust pose), *Ardha-Matsyendrasana* (lateral twist), *Makarasana* (crocodile pose), *Shavasana* (corpse pose), *Pranayam* (breath control) and *Meditation.* An experienced yoga teacher can change the order of these practices depending on the condition and need of the patient.

A typical yoga session begins (preferably in the mornings) with light limbering exercises on an empty stomach and after evacuating the bowels, followed by pranayam and meditation. It concludes with Shavasana. Yoga improves breathing, leading to improved circulation. Good circulation is crucial to all phases of immune reaction. Immune cells travel through the blood stream and lymphatic fluid to patrol the body for invaders. Since not every helper T-cell can recognize every invader, it is necessary to assist helper T-cells in getting around to all their checkpoints. Yoga asanas that squeeze, soak, and strengthen the organs of immune surveillance (skin, gastrointestinal tract, respiratory tract) also promote strong defenses at these important body frontiers. See the graphic presentation above and for better results join yoga classes in your vicinity.

SHANKHAPRAKSHALANA is an effective technique to cleanse the alimentary canal. In this, the patient drinks about 10 to 20 glasses of warm saline water, repeating five asanas given along-side eight times each. This *kriya* takes at least two hours and should be done strictly under expert guidance. It helps relax the valves from mouth to the anus region expelling the feacal matter and cleansing the system fully. Specific for diabetes and other chronic diseases like acidity, ulcers, colitis, tuberculosis. Anaemic patients, thin and wiry

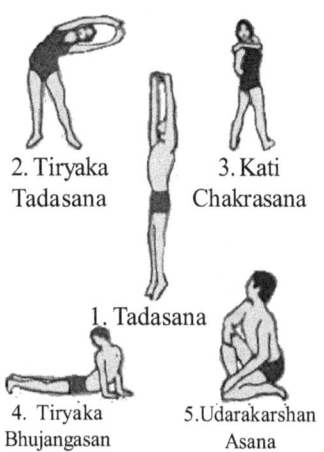

2. Tiryaka
Tadasana

3. Kati
Chakrasana

1. Tadasana

4. Tiryaka
Bhujangasan

5.Udarakarshan
Asana

persons start putting on weight after this cleansing process. Additional practices to be done with this are: *Kunjal Kriya and Jala Neti.*

Like the Sun does not fail to rise and illuminate the Earth, similarly, Yoga does not fail to effect cure, provided, you have got the sense and patience.

DR. LEO REBELLO's AIDS VACCINES

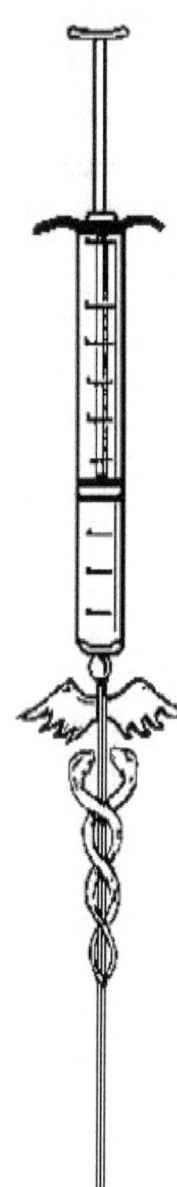

1.. In the case of AIDS the diseased part basically is the blood. As such, we can prepare a highly effective nosode (homeopathic vaccine) from the AIDS patient's blood and try it universally as a prophylactic as well as a cure. And since AIDS symptoms are not universally alike but highly individualistic with the HIV mutating in various forms, this researcher feels and advocates Auto Blood Therapy. Take a HIV+ patient's blood sample, prepare a homeopathic dilution of it and administer the same back as a vaccine.

2.. Likewise, AIDS patient's urine taken/potentised and given over a period of time, to be decided individually. Ten drops of urine of the concerned patient mixed in 90 drops of rectified spirit can make 1X medicine to be used by the patient.

3.. AIDS patient's blood mixed with pulsatilla or phosphorus mother tincture, shaken well and given according to the need and observation will also work wonders.

Why part of the Aids Vaccine fund cannot be made available to test the above proven concepts rather than groping in the dark? But no, the medical mafia does not want that to happen because the economies of many western nations will simply collapse the day three lethal industries are closed down, namely, the Arms, Drugs and synthetic Food Industries.

VEGGIE VACCINES

Scientists are turning fruits and vegetables into drugs, vaccines and antibiotics. One of the first to hit the market is a potato vaccine designed to protect against a form of gastroenteritis called Norwalk (caused by seafood) and E-coli. Then there is a banana vaccine. Genetically altered half a banana will protect children from polio, cholera and other diseases. Also on the anvil are malaria and cancer vaccines. In another ten years, if the experiment succeeds, these edible vaccines will be delivered through food.

The potatoes, fresh from the greenhouse of Prof. Charles Arntzen at Cornell University in New York, are part of a revolution that is turning bananas, corn, beans, tomatoes and many other crops into drugs, vaccines and antibiotics. Scientists are currently altering the genetic profile of these plants so that they can grow proteins and antibodies that will fight off or prevent diseases in the humans that eat them. The technology of edible vaccines is relatively simple. A gene is taken from the bacteria or virus and mixed into the genetic make-up of the plant, which develops a 'foreign' antigen or protein in response to the presence of a new gene.

When the patients eat the genetically engineered fruit or vegetable, their immune system will detect the antigen and produce antibodies to fight it. In this way, the body would be immunised. So, when the real virus or bacteria comes along, the immune system can repel it because it already has the antigen to recognise it. These Veggie Vaccines will also not have the animal diseases crossing to human beings.

Let us hope that these genetically altered potatoes will not make our skulls grow out of shape or our penises like bananas! Genetically altered chickens, have already made chickens out of men. Why cannot you eat God's own fruits? It is, as the Bible says, when Satan thought he was wiser than his Creator, all hell let lose. Present day doctors and scientists are playing God (or Satan?) with the patients and the world.

DR. LEO REBELLO'S
TEN HEALTH COMMANDMENTS

When God, the finest manufacturer of this intricate body and all that is there, gave you this beautiful body, he also gave you a guarantee card of 100 years of fault-free service. But you have misplaced that card and I am going to help you today to find that card and live to be Healthy Hundred. Like Moses gave Ten Commandments, following which the society can run smoothly, the ten commandments of health devised by me, if followed without compromise, are guaranteed to help you complete a century.

1. Eat twice a day only, preferably raw.
Ayurveda (the science of life) recorded thousands of years ago that one should not eat more than twice a day. It enjoins on you to eat a good breakfast, because that is the principal meal of the day, and finish your dinner before sunset. There is also a very apt saying: one who eats once is a *Yogi* (self-realized), one who eats twice is a *Bhogi* (glutton) and one who eats thrice is a *Rogi* (diseased)!

Diet is your destiny. Many dishes, many diseases. More people die due to overeating than due to malnutrition. But overeating statistics are distributed as deaths due to Obesity, High BP, Diabetes, Cancers, etc.

Food sustains life. But as epitomised in the idiom 'not by bread alone', it is not the only thing that keeps the life going. Coronaries, our lifelines, need fresh air, pure water and fruits. Not fried, fatty and fast food. The ultimate Truth is that life stops when wastes from the ingested food and from the thoughts assimilated are not discharged or expelled regularly and in the quantity equal to intake. Don't indulge and you won't bulge. With increasing age, Wisdom should increase not the weight.

2. Drink minimum 8 glasses of water to wash out toxins.
On an average, we lose 3 litres of fluid daily from the body – by way of urination, perspiration, spitting, etc. The human body is made up of 67% of water. Unless this balance is maintained by adequate intake of water,

the blood will be surcharged with wastes and diseased matter. It will then turn acidic, thick and will not circulate easily. Healthy blood stream should be 70% alkaline and 30% acidic. But because of our wrong habits, this ratio is in inverse proportion. Hence diseases.

Less intake of water will lead to constipation, acidity, ulceration, pressure on the kidneys, skin diseases, varicose veins, heart problems, obesity, loss of libido and hosts of other diseases. Hence, it is very essential that you drink adequate water (repeat water), not liquid. Because liquid would include tea, coffee, liquor, aerated waters, etc., which are in themselves harmful to health.

3. Meditate twice a day, for good mental health and stress-free life. Tension needs urgent attention to avoid hypertension. Meditation is like going on a holiday, daily. Meditation will help you to relax, to unwind, to improve, to smile, to be happy, to be stress-free, and to lead a fuller life.

The difference between Prayer and Meditation is: In prayer you talk to God. In Meditation, you listen to Him. As such, meditation is far superior to prayer and going to temples, mosques or churches to meet God.

Meditate ten minutes in the morning and again ten minutes in the night. Too long a meditation itself becomes counter productive. In the morning remind yourself that you have been given one more day of opportunity. The darkness of night (as also from your life) has vanished. Thank God for one more day of opportunity, for there is no guarantee when you go to sleep that you will ever open your eyes! In the evening when you meditate, recall whether you have done anything wrong, willy-nilly. If so, give auto-suggestion that this will not recur again. "To err is human, but to rise after a fall is manly and glorious".

4. Exercise for minimum 15 minutes daily and stand and walk upright. For we have about 700 muscles in our body, including our Heart (which is the strongest muscle or pump). These muscles, unless exercised regularly, become weak and sluggish. They atrophy, they become the storehouse of toxins, deposits and fats. The body and internal organs degenerate, all kinds of 'dis-eases' set in and one ages prematurely. Exercise helps you to keep your youthfulness and vigour.

Surya Namaskar is the easiest form of exercise. It helps you to remove both 'mental' and 'gastrointestinal' constipation. It is the complete exercise which helps you to breathe out and discharge poisons which inhibit life. You could also cycle, swim, skip, jog or play rugged games like tennis, football or hockey, participate in aerobics, dancercises, etc. But please avoid weight-lifting, power-lifting exercises. They stunt your growth, make you slow and reduce your life span because of burn out.

5. Fast once a week to give rest to your vital organs.
All internal organs are vital organs. They work incessantly. Many a time you overload them beyond their capacity by various excesses. Fasting will help them rest and recuperate. By fasting one day once a week, I mean, full 24 hours of liquid intake in which only following items are permitted – warm water, citric fruit juices, fresh buttermilk (without salt or sugar), coconut water. No milk, no tea, no coffee, no liquor, no aerated waters are permitted during fasting.

To the above five main commandments add the following five more commandments:-

6. Do not smoke, or take drugs, or drink alcohol. For, too much of a tasty toast brings out tummy and troubles.

7. Do not gamble or cheat. Gambling is a psychological affliction, which has ruined many. When you cheat others, you cheat yourself, you cheat God.

8. Sex is not bad. In fact, natural sex (not forced, mechanical or bought) is one of the best exercises for good physical and mental health and spiritual wellbeing.

9. Sleep well - body requires 6 to 8 hours of night sleep for good physical and mental health. Melatonin produced during the night sleep will delay the ageing process. But do not take sleeping pills, for they are habit forming and some day you may overdose and sleep permanently. During long flights, especially the night flights, sleep is very important to get over jet lag. Also, keep drinking fruit juices and water to avoid dehydration.

10. And come what may, go on smiling. Smile not only has a therapeutic effect on the person who keeps on smiling, but also on the person receiving it. Like coming of the Sun the darkness of the night disappears, with smile troubles disappear, pain eases out, relaxation which descends improves breathing, which in turn help repair the internal organs. A smile is contagious. Why not spread a contagion?

After reading this you are sure to ask me: if we cannot do all these 'good things' in life, then why live at all? Well, I live to enjoy nature's bounty, to see rainbow colours, to hear birds sing while flying into the limitless azure sky, to realize my potential, to smile, to spread happiness, to lead a full life and vibrant health and to make the world a better place to live in. Follow my above commandments if you wish to enjoy good health throughout.

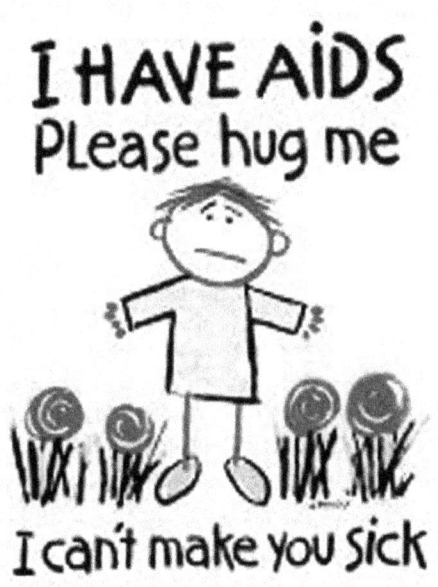

ADDENDUM

HUMANISM IN MEDICINE
(Text of speech delivered by Dr. Leo Rebello
in Durban, South Africa, on 16 July, 2000)

Today's morning papers say that the American tobacco giants Malbro have been fined equivalent of R1000 million for endangering people's lives for suppressing information that tobacco causes cancer.

Likewise, Glaxo – the transnational pharmaceutical giant, which recently reduced the price of AZT by 90% to capture the African market (this is called dumping strategy) should also be fined for promoting AZT, a carcinogen, as an AIDS cure and endangering the present and future generations.

Hereby, I am inviting physicians, healers, researchers, human rights activists and AIDS patients worldwide to join a growing consortium of people and professionals committed to resolving the 'man-made' tragedy of AIDS through practical, innovative efforts. **Our goals are:-**
* Broaden the scope of current AIDS research by designing and implementing clinical research unlimited by the HIV paradigm and the overuse of health-compromising chemical drugs.
* Identify non-toxic, health-enhancing treatments that can be economically applied on a global level.
* Construct an international network of peer support for HIV+ and AIDS diagnosed persons who elect to use alternative therapies or decline current faulty standards of care.
* Create a referral network of medical and alternative practitioners who honour the right and the ability of HIV/AIDS diagnosed persons to achieve and maintain optimum health, using non-toxic therapies.
* Establish a human rights advocacy commission and legal advisory partnership to assist HIV positives, whose civil and human rights are violated; who are denied rights to informed choice with regard to testing and treatment; who are threatened with loss of custody of children or employment due to decisions to forego AIDS drug treatments.

* Grow a PR network of authors, journalists, publishers, broadcasters and entertainers committed to global promotion of alternative and sensible voices on AIDS.

* Raise funds untethered from interests that conflict with goals of health and health freedom.

* Unite to make South Africa/Asia and the world AIDS-free. From Aids Scare, which destroys people, families, economies, let us work for Aids Care.

In a democratic world, why should we tolerate medical hegemony? Why should there be apartheid in medicine? I am here, like Mikhail Gorbachev to introduce perestroika (a new thinking) in health sector. I appeal to you to throw off your sunglasses and see the bright reality. I appeal to you to come out of your tiny pond of ignorance and swim into the limitless ocean of knowledge. Let us talk of Holistic Health. Let us bring some Humanism into Medicine.

W.H.O. & TRADITIONAL MEDICINE
Salient features of the Consultations
with Dr. Leo Rebello's sharp comments

In July 1990, World Health Organisation conducted Consultations on Aids and Traditional Medicine in Francistown, Botswana. I have a full report of the said meeting and give below some extracts from WHO publication (no. WHO/TRM/GPA/90.1). **I have given my comments wherever necessary and they are highlighted for your consideration.**

From Page 3 - Introduction Chapter
In 1976, the World Health Assembly acknowledged the potential value of traditional medicine in expanding health services by calling attention to the manpower reserve constituted by traditional health practitioners (resolution WHA29.72). In the following year, a World Health Assembly resolution (WHA30.49) urged countries to utilize their traditional systems of medicine. Another resolution was passed in 1978, in which the Organization was called upon to develop a comprehensive approach to the subject of medicinal plants (WHA31.33). Nine years later, in 1987, the Fortieth World Health Assembly reaffirmed the main points of the earlier resolutions,

as well as related recommendations made at the International Conference on Primary Health Care, held in Alma-Ata, USSR, in 1978 (WHA40.33).

The Forty-first World Health Assembly drew attention to the Chiang Mai Declaration (1988): "Save Plants that Save Lives" and endorsed the call for international cooperation and coordination to establish a basis for the conservation of medicinal plants, in order to ensure that adequate quantities be available for the use of future generations (resolution WHA41.19).

In 1989, a resolution was passed (WHA42.43) that recalled earlier resolutions on traditional medicine, traditional health practitioners, and traditional remedies and affirmed that together they constitute a comprehensive approach to the utilization of medicinal plants in the health services.

Contd. from Page 6 of the Report
2.1 Guidelines for formulating policies on training, research, and ethical issues in traditional medicine and AIDS
Countries should themselves decide which types of traditional practitioners they would want to involve in their national AIDS prevention, control, and care activities. While it is important to distinguish between different types of practitioners, it is understood that all types of traditional health practitioners recognized by their communities may well have important roles to play in AIDS prevention, counseling, and care in community leadership.

(In India, we have six recognised systems of medicine, namely, Ayurveda, Naturopathy, Homeopathy, Siddha, Unani and Allopathy. But the Alternative Medical Practitioner is always given a step motherly treatment, even though India gave to the world Ayurveda, Acupuncture, Yoga, etc.)

2.1.1 The purpose of a policy on traditional medicine is:
(a) to protect the patient from substandard care;
(b) to recognize the role of traditional health practitioners and define their rights, privileges, and responsibilities as health care providers;

(c) to correct the serious neglect in the education and training (including continuing education) of traditional practitioners and in research on the effectiveness of their practices.

2.1.3 A policy on traditional medicine should provide guidelines for the following major areas: legislation and regulation; education and training; research and development; ethical issues; and allocation of financial and other resources.

Special training of traditional health practitioners for their participation in certain primary health care programmes must be emphasized. Appropriate entry points for their involvement in primary health care activities could be:
* oral rehydration therapy;
* traditional midwives for primary health care centres;
* family planning programmes;
* control of sexually transmitted diseases and AIDS;
* integrated AIDS and family planning programmes;
* endemic disease control such as of leprosy and tuberculosis;
* expanded programme on immunization;
(Why hazardous allopathic immunization programme is being forced by World Health Organization on unsuspecting people? Why not try homeopathic vaccines or veggie vaccines?)
* nutritional education;
* breast-feeding;
* elaboration of national traditional medicine pharmacopoeia;
* needs assessment through KABP (knowledge, attitudes, beliefs and practices) surveys and AIDS;
* collection and dissemination of information and simple statistics on health care.

Contd. from Page 8 of the Report
(d) To ensure that the practice of traditional medicine be respectable, * fundamental human rights must be codified and adhered to. These should include :
* protection of the individual;
* confidentiality in practice;

* informed consent in studies and drug trials;
* avoidance of prejudice against patients (e.g. those with AIDS, other STDs, leprosy);
* respect for the dead;
* respect for proprietary rights and intellectual property;
* adequate compensation (for practitioners' services, malpractice suits);
* promotion of national resource regeneration and conservation.

* (The most fundamental human right is Right to Health. It is as important as Right to Life. But this is being violated brazenly by WHO and even by the democratic governments of the world when they make chlorination of drinking water, iodisation of salt and deleterious allopathic vaccinations compulsory or when they force even carcinogenic AZT onto pregnant mothers. When inadequately tested drugs are marketed and dumped in Afro-Asian markets, when HIV-infected blood from Africa is clandestinely supplied to Asian countries to increase the number of AIDS patients, when without consent AIDS vaccine trials take place, when some mercenary American pharmaceutical companies or individuals corner the patent for turmeric, neem and other medicinal plants which have been used for centuries as home remedies, what fundamental right WHO is talking of? To what use are its pious sentiments when its actions speak contrary to the human welfare? Will WHO reply to these straight questions and democratic governments address them?)

Contd. from Page 10 of the Report
2.2.6 An outline of ways to involve traditional health practitioners in national AIDS programmes

There is no simple or single approach to involving traditional health practitioners in national AIDS programmes; however, this should be based on mutual trust and collaboration between all health care workers.

(a) Where there is formal recognition of traditional health practitioners, with established specific organizational structures, they should be represented on national, provincial, and district AIDS committees. This could be an initial step towards recognizing their role and soliciting their support in national AIDS programmes. (Can WHO show as to how many countries have done this?)

Contd..from Page 11 of the Report
(i) There should be a provision in the budgets of AIDS control programmes specifically for the active involvement of traditional health practitioners in AIDS prevention and control. When traditional health practitioners first begin to participate in these programmes, it would be necessary to make funds available for a number of activities, including seminars and the production of education materials, and for the remuneration of national and provincial focal points/coordinators, since they will devote most of their time to organizing their members and developing and coordinating different identified activities **(Nothing has been done in this regard too).**

2.3 Identification of target groups of traditional health practitioners for training, development of training methodology, and identification of training materials

2.3.1 Efforts should be made to train all categories of traditional health practitioners in AIDS prevention and control, whether or not they are part of the formal health system. They will, in turn, become trainers for their client population, thus promoting a multiplier effect.

Contd. from Page 12 of the Report
2.4 Identification of research priorities
Research priorities are defined in the context of the traditional health practitioner's role in the prevention and control of AIDS. These include:
* traditional health practitioners' perceptions of AIDS (diagnosis, prevention, treatment, patient care, and cure);
* he community's perception of the traditional health practitioner's role and activities in AIDS prevention and control;

Contd. from Page 13 of the Report
* counseling techniques of the traditional health practitioners;
* ways to promote cooperation of traditional health practitioners in scientific research on traditional medicine and AIDS;

* the best ways to inform traditional health practitioners and the general public about AIDS;
* ways to involve traditional health practitioners in epidemiological surveys and surveillance.

Present research policies in most countries do not reflect the role of traditional medicine in the delivery of health care. New research and development policies could greatly assist institutions in addressing the critical problem now being faced throughout the world of controlling and preventing the spread of AIDS.

3.. RECOMMENDATIONS
In recognition of the vital role that traditional health practitioners have to play in national AIDS prevention and control activities, the consultation made the following recommendations to countries:

3.1 Policy and Legislation
3.1.1 All countries should formulate a national policy on traditional medicine. Such a policy should be aimed at improving the overall health and welfare of the population within the framework of national primary health care programmes.

3.1.2 A national traditional medicine research policy should be formulated and implemented by a multidisciplinary traditional medicine research council that includes traditional health practitioners among its members.

3.1.3 Countries should consider establishing policies that would guarantee the intellectual property and patent rights of individuals and institutions involved in research and development of new drugs from traditional remedies. Such a policy should indicate how income potentially arising from these discoveries should be distributed.

3.1.4 A policy should be formulated to provide adequate funding from national budgets to ensure the active involvement of traditional health practitioners. External sources of funding should only be considered as secondary or supplemental resources to the normal government expenditure.

3.1.5 A well-defined policy should be followed by legislation that defines and standardizes basic elements of prevalent traditional medicine practices. Such a legislation should clearly state the rights, responsibilities, and privileges of traditional health practitioners. The legislation should also be directed towards the conservation and rational utilization of traditional medical resources, including vegetables, animal, and mineral products, upon which many traditional health practitioners depend. There should also be legislation to ensure equity in the distribution of income generated from the sale of drugs developed from traditional sources.

Contd. from Page 14 of the Report
3.3 Research

3.3.2 Technology transfer should be an integral part of any research agreement with foreign investigators/institutions, so that national research capabilities can be strengthened.

3.3.5 Multidisciplinary, action-oriented research should be undertaken as the best means of promoting traditional medicine and utilizing traditional health practitioners in primary health care, especially in the prevention and control of AIDS and HIV infections. Involvement of local personnel in research teams (e.g. traditional health practitioners, community health workers, nurses, botanists, etc.) should be encouraged. Feedback of research results to all personnel and institutions involved in the project should be ensured.

(How about allocating atleast 25% of the total research grant to alternative medicine without strings attached? Also, why should WHO insist that the alternative medical practitioners should follow the dubious research protocols of modern medicine? Why can't WHO study the time-tested research protocol of Alternative Medicine? Why does not WHO or World Bank or America allocate a part of Vaccine-grant to Veggie Vaccines, Homeopathic Vaccines, and other Vaccines projects? How many standard publications of Alternative Medicine have been published by WHO? How many conferences are held on Alternative Medicine vis-à-vis the

Conferences on Modern Medicine? Why, in the International AIDS Conferences, Alternative Medical Practitioners are not given opportunities to present their research work during main tracks? Why are they always sidelined? Why Alternative Medical Practitioners are not nominated for Nobel Prize in Medicine, even though there is a provision in Nobel's Will to that effect? Of the total budget of WHO, how much is used for the promotion of Alternative Medicine? Even though, 80% of the world population depends on Traditional and Natural Medicine, why not even 20% funds earmarked for health are allocated to them? Is WHO really the World Health Organization or is it a Federation of Pharmaceutical, Petroleum and Chemical Companies? What justice, equity, fair play are we talking of? WHO have you got answers to these pertinent questions?)

BAN ALL HIV ANTIBODY TESTING

HIV testing is non-specific, non-standardized and unreliable. How can one possibly identify a virus from antibodies? When HI virus itself is missing what antibodies? ELISA and Western Blot tests for HIV cross-react with over 60 known medical conditions and illnesses (see below) according to Christine Johnson and other researchers. Therefore, labelling patients with HIV positive and stigmatizing them is not proper. That leads to suicides and iatrogenic genocide due to carcinogenic anti-retrovirals as part of the double-edged government weapon to reduce population.

* Acute viral infections, DNA viral infections
* Alcoholic liver diseases
* Anti-carbohydrate antibodies
* Anti-collagen antibodies
* Anti-hepatitis A IgM (antibody)
* Blood transfusions
* Epstein-Barr virus
* Flu vaccination
* Hemophilia
* Hemodialysis/renal failure
* Hepatitis and Hepatitis B vaccination

* Herpes simplex I and II
* Hyperbilirubinemia
* Leprosy
* Malaria
* Malignant neoplasms (cancers)
* Naturally-occuring antibodies
* Organ transplantation
* Other retroviruses
* Passive immunization : receipt of gamma globulin or immune globulin
* Pregnancy in multiparous women
* Recent viral infection or exposure to viral vaccines
* Renal failure
* Renal transplantation
* Rheumatoid arthritis
* Stevens-Johnson syndrome
* 'Sticky' blood (in Africans)
* Tetanus vaccination
* Tuberculosis
* Upper respiratory tract infection (cold or flu)

DOCTORS, DRUGS & DEVILS

The person most likely to kill you is not a burglar, a mugger, a deranged relative or a drunken driver. The person most likely to kill you is your doctor. In India, a doctor is called Yama's younger brother. Yama according to Hindu mythology is a god of death.

Here is an apt Sanskrit commentary
Vaidyaraj namastubhyam
Yamaraj sahodar
Yamastu harati pranan
Vaidya pranan dhanani cha

Doctor, I salute thee
For being the brother of Yama
Yama, however, only takes life
You take life as well as wealth.

Here are some statistics from America which shows how dangerous is the medical establishment : 150,000 to 300,000 Americans are injured or killed each year because of medical negligence (i.e., mistreated diseases, surgeries, drug reactions, misprescribed drugs) —Wall Street Journal, January 13, 1993. Iatrogenic diseases, generally defined as diseases that result from a physician's action or in response to a drug, are believed to be a major problem in terms of morbidity and hospital expense. "Over a million patients are injured in hospitals each year, and approximately 180,000 die annually as a result of these injuries.* Therefore, the iatrogenic injury rate dwarfs the annual automobile accident mortality of 45,000 and accounts for more deaths than all other accidents combined." JAMA, July 5, 1995, 274 : 29-34.

* [Note : This is roughly equivalent to three jumbo jets loaded with passengers - crashing and killing everyone aboard - every two days! Would you fly if the airline industry had that kind of record?]

Stanford University doctors compared the effects of chemotherapy with 'doing nothing' in patients with slow-growing tumors of the lymph nodes. The patients whose treatment was deferred for years did just as well as the patients who immediately received expensive and unpleasant chemotherapy. 19 of the 83 (or 23%) experienced spontaneous remission lasting four months to six years. A 1992 review of the study in the New England Journal of Medicine concluded: "...deferring treatment may allow for spontaneous regression of the disease." Chemotherapy and radiation can increase the risk of developing a second cancer by up to 100 times, according to Dr. Samuel Epstein. – Congressional Record, September 9, 1987.

Out of every 1,000 American women getting mammograms done each year between the ages of 40 and 50, 345 will receive false positive results, often with unnecessary intervention as the result. — New England Journal of Medicine, February 11, 1993. About 90% of the patients who visit doctors have conditions that will either improve on their own or are out of reach of modern medicine's ability to solve. — New England Journal of Medicine, February 7, 1991.

In 1976 in Bogota, Colombia, doctors went on strike. During a 52-day period the death rate went down 35%. In Los Angeles in 1976, doctors went on strike to protest increasing costs of malpractice insurance. The death rate decreased by 18%. When the strike ended, the death rate returned to pre-strike proportions. In Israel in 1973, during a month-long strike, the death rate dropped 50%. The last time the death rate had been that low was when there was a doctors' strike 20 years before. - **Confessions of a Medical Heretic, Robert Menndelsohn, M.D.** Harvard researchers studied hospital records from the state of New York over a one-year period. They estimated that more than 13,000 New Yorkers were killed and 2,500 permanently disabled due to medical care. More than 51% of the deaths were blamed on negligence. — New England Journal of Medicine, February 7, 1991. During 1983-1992, between 90,000 to 110,000 Americans died from reactions to prescription drugs, but no one died due to herbs.

Glaxo Wellcome Plc, according to Reuter report of August 14, 2000, confirmed that its HIV treatment drug Ziagen can spark serious and sometimes fatal reactions in patients, but said that the problems were known. An unknown number of patients have died as a result of Ziagen, which was launched in the United States and Europe in 1998. Glaxo said about four percent of patients were susceptible to hypersensitivity of this drug. But the company spokesman skirted the issue by saying that they had kept doctors and patients informed of the possible side-effects, even before the drug was licensed. Glaxo's HIV drugs — from the late 1980s Retrovir (AZT) to its most recent ones, Ziagen and Agenerase — together account for a third of the market, and their sales are growing.

AZT for AIDS is a known carcinogen which inhibits bone-marrow production, which in turn necessitates continual blood tranfusion for many patients. Yet Glaxo markets it inspite of known dangers. Since Thabo Mbeiki, South African President, refused to prescribe it to pregnant mothers, Glaxo reduced the price by 90% for South Africa, saying poor Africa cannot afford and hence as a social responsibility and humanitarian consideration they were reducing the price. That means even at 10%, Glaxo can make profit. This lethal drug till recently was available in India for Rs.40,000 a month per patient. Now, because of government subsidy, the cost is Rs.25,000. Subsidy for whom?

When profits speak, can logic follow? Alas, when will the HIV/AIDS patients realize this sinister game of the medical mafia? As Dom Martin wrote in his letter to the Editor of San Francisco Chronicle on July 13, 2000: "To profit from disease is to exploit human misery, and unless this franchise of greed is reversed with unconditional humanism, the pain and suffering of the overwhelming majority shall continue to be the cauldron of unconscionable wealth for corporations and the affluent, and in time, equate their guilt to the very sins of the Holocaust".

WHY AZT SHOULD BE BANNED

Now read what a HIV positive mother, whose child is negative, Christine Maggiore has to say in her book aptly titled WHAT IF EVERYTHING YOU THOUGHT YOU KNEW ABOUT AIDS WAS WRONG? The book has been published by the American Foundation for AIDS Alternatives, of which I am one of the advisors.

AZT is not a new drug. It was not created for the treatment of AIDS and is not an antiviral. AZT is a chemical compound that was developed as a potential chemotherapy treatment for cancer in 1964. It was soon abandoned because of its lethal effects on rats. Prior to the first AIDS drug trials in 1986, AZT had never been administered to human beings.

Chemotherapy works by killing all growing cells in the body. Many cancer patients do not survive chemotherapy due to its destructive effects on the immune system and intestines. Because of the damage it causes, chemotherapy is never used as a preventive for cancer, and is only administered for very limited amounts of time.

Since cancer is a condition of persistently growing cells, AZT was designed to prevent the formation of new cells by blocking development of DNA chains. In 1964, experiments with AZT on mice with cancer showed that AZT was so effective in destroying healthy growing cells that the mice

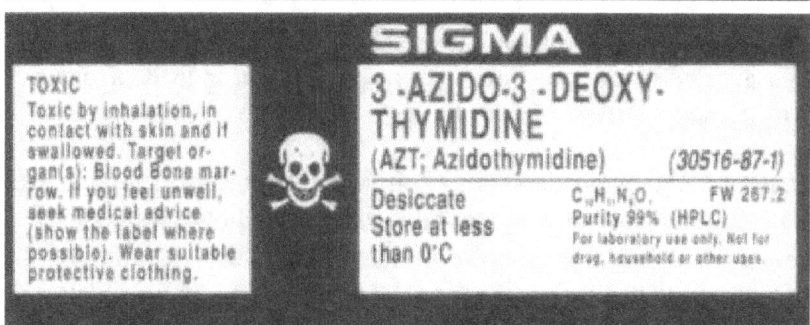

SIGMA

3-AZIDO-3-DEOXY-THYMIDINE

(AZT; Azidothymidine)   (30516-87-1)

Desiccate $C_{10}H_{13}N_5O_4$ FW 267.2
Store at less   Purity 99% (HPLC)
than 0°C   For laboratory use only. Not for drug, household or other uses.

This label has appeared on bottles containing as little as 25 milligrams, a small fraction ($\frac{1}{20}$ to $\frac{1}{60}$) of a patient's daily prescribed dose of 500 to 1,500 mg

died of extreme toxicity. As a result, AZT was shelved and no patent was ever filed. Twenty years later, the pharmaceutical company Burroughs Wellcome (now Glaxo-Wellcome) began a campaign to re-market AZT as an anti-HIV drug based on the idea that AZT would block the formation of HIV DNA chains. Glaxo-Wellcome won FDA approval for AZT as an AIDS treatment after one highly flawed study of only four months duration. Approval of this extremely toxic chemotherapy for use by AIDS patients was based on information which suggested that AZT raised levels of T cells and therefore delayed the onset of AIDS indicator diseases. The rise noted in T cells was interpreted as evidence that AZT eradicated HIV in T cells, a concept for which there is no scientific proof. Although the study was halted before any long-term effects of AZT were known, proponents established that standard treatment with AZT should be continuous and lifelong.

A multitude of independent studies conducted before and after FDA approval, including the Concorde study – the largest (1,749 subjects) and longest (three years in duration) study on AZT – determined that AZT increases T cell counts only moderately and briefly without improving health and that it does not delay onset of AIDS indicator diseases.

The brief rise in T cells noted when AZT use is initiated is due to the toxic nature of the drug and to the blood system's response to the destruction of bone marrow. As AZT destroys bone marrow, the blood system attempts to correct this depletion by overproducing T cells, often creating more new T cells than the number found in a patient's blood prior to beginning treatment. But as the source of these new T cells – the bone marrow – is killed off by AZT, the level of T cells drops lower, ultimately causing complete destruction of the immune system. Individual tolerance to and absorption of AZT determine length of survival on this toxic compound.

Following recommendations for "early intervention," one-third to one-half of HIV positives who develop AIDS do so only after taking AZT. Independent studies have shown that AZT actually accelerates clinical decline and decreases quality of life, at times even causing death before any AIDS-defining illnesses appear – an occurrence officially described as "death without any preceding AIDS-defining event".

The concept of "HIV mutation" has become a popular explanation for the fall in T cells observed in patients treated with AZT. Promoters of the mutation hypothesis assert that the positive effects of AZT are diminished by mutant strains of HIV that become resistant to the drug. There is, however, no scientific evidence to substantiate their claim.

In addition to destroying T cells, B cells and the red blood cells that carry oxygen throughout the body, AZT and other nucleoside analog drugs destroy the kidneys, liver, intestines, muscle tissue, and the central nervous system. Nucleoside analog drugs also interfere with the activities of mitochondria, the sub-cellular particles that are the energy factories of every living cell in the body. Mitochondria contain their own DNA which makes them vulnerable to the effects of nucleoside analogs.

Epivir (3TC), Zerit (D4T), Hivid (ddC) and Videx (ddI) are all nucleoside analog drugs prescribed to HIV positives as "antivirals." All are modeled after AZT, and all work in the same manner.

B cells: One of two principal types of lymphocytes (white blood cells). B cells are transformed into plasma cells that secrete immunoglobulins or antibodies that destroy invading microorganisms. The protective effect of immunoglobulins is called humoral immunity.

Nucleoside analog: A synthetic compound similar to one of the components of DNA or RNA. Nucleoside analogs such as AZT act as artificial caps to DNA chains which prevent real DNA units from being added. For this reason these drugs are often referred to as DNA chain terminators.

AIDS BY PRESCRIPTION

The following conditions are caused by nucleoside analog drugs (AZT, ddl, ddC, D4T and 3TC). Conditions followed by a bullet (•) are official AIDS-defining illnesses:

Anemia (requiring transfusions)	Lymphoma (cancer) •
Birth defects	Muscle wasting •
Diarrhea •	Nausea
Dementia •	Neuropathy
Fertility impairment	Pancreatitis
Granulocytbpenia	**Pancytopenia**
Hair loss	Seizures
Headaches	Skin discolorations
Liver damage	Spontaneous abortion
Loss of appetite	T cell depletion •

Those who say that HIV is a deadly virus, also claim that it can easily be destroyed by:

Boiling – inactivated in 1 second.
Ethanol – 70 per cent, or 700 mg/ltr solution.
Household bleach – 1 per cent solution.
Hydrogen peroxide – 3 per cent solution.
Isopropyl alcohol – 35 per cent solution.
So, why this panic reaction?

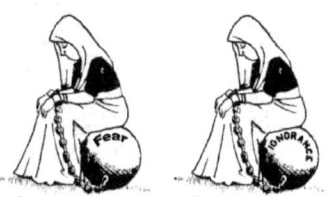

of HIV-AIDS and other Alternatives Available.

David Ho(ax) and his lethal cocktails
Celia Farber's stunning article circulated on 13 February 2000
by cinex@cedbom.ilbom.ernet.in

It's telling, and perfectly symbolic that when AIDS researcher David Ho's face appeared on the cover of Time magazine as Man of the Year, 1996, you couldn't see his eyes. Instead, a colorful swirl meant to represent HIV filled his glasses. George Orwell used precisely this image-a man whose eyes are gone, whose glasses have been filled with the refracting light of his ideology - to convey the triumph of politics over truth in his famous essay Politics and the English Language.

Ho, the then newly appointed director of the Aaron Diamond AIDS Research Center in New York, was suddenly catapulted to a degree of fame, and gave him an oracular power over the press and the AIDS community. The son of Chinese immigrants, he was a man obsessed with HIV, and his vision was to bomb it with not one drug, or two, but a literal hail. He popularized the idea that HIV, far from being the cryptic, latent, quiet virus most researchers thought it was - was in fact 'replicating furiously', from the very moment of infection. The immune system, he wrongly surmised, would collapse before the furiously replicating virus. He was a man of simple concepts, and the one that would alter history went like this: hit hard, hit early.

Ho's bogus experiment, which spread to media around the world before it was ever completed, was to knock back HIV to the point of being 'undetectable', then take the patients off the 'cocktail' of drugs, with HIV banished for good. His recipe for a cure was to create a blitzkrieg of chemicals – a mixture of old AIDS drugs like AZT with the new class of drugs waiting in the pipeline called 'protease inhibitors' - to annihilate HIV in the bloodstream. Protease inhibitors had been researched since the early 90s by the major drug companies, several of which came close to abandoning the effort because the drugs did not work against HIV.

David Ho, Time magazine gushed, "fundamentally changed the way scientists looked at the AIDS virus... His pioneering experiments with protease inhibitors helped clarify how the virus ultimately overwhelms the immune system... Mathematical models suggest that patients caught early enough might be virus-free within two or three years". David Ho, Time concluded, delivered "what may be the most important fact about AIDS: it is not invincible".

Based largely on a single paper- Ho's 1995 paper- protease inhibitors received lightening-quick FDA approval and poured onto the market. The mass media declared AIDS to be "over"! No body looked at the question mark lurking overhead. A new euphoria filled the air, and David Ho spawned a multibillion-dollar drug industry. Amidst the excitement, something was overlooked. Ho's mathematical model was wrong.

The phone rang late one night and Shawn O'Hearn, 33, a San Francisco HIV prevention worker, answered it. It was an old friend, a successful dancer who, although he had tested positive for HIV, had remained in perfect health. Following the advice of the nation's leading AIDS organizations, he had begun taking a cocktail of drugs including protease inhibitors, even though he didn't have any symptoms of disease. Four weeks later, he suffered a stroke. "I am paralyzed, Shawn", he told O'Hearn. He'll never dance or even walk again.

This is not a rare story. Such tragedies are seen as an inevitable 'side effect' of a drug regimen so punishing that an entire surveillance system has been put in place to ensure that people stick to it. There are computer chips embedded in bottle caps that record the date and time of each opening. There are beepers, support groups, buddy systems, observation centers where patients take the drugs while being watched, and even groups of AIDS professionals who infiltrate people's social networks to enlist them to help promote and dispense the drugs. They call it 'treatment compliance', and it has largely replaced 'Safe Sex' as the core social imperative of the AIDS industry. The goal is to get as many HIV-positive people on the drugs as possible, whether they are sick or healthy. And to keep them on them, through debilitating ill effects, which are dismissed as a small price to pay for the benefit of lowering the amount of virus in the blood. But now, four years after the initial AIDS cocktail drug hype erupted, this fake experiment is fast turning into a nightmare for millions.

"I started to notice that more and more friends, young people, were suffering these mysterious strokes and heart attacks", says O'Hearn, a member of the HIV Prevention Planning Council in San Francisco. "They are listed as AIDS deaths. But those are not AIDS deaths, those are drug deaths". San Francisco is a crucible for the new schism in the AIDS community. The city's AIDS culture has long been characterized and dominated by the mainstream organisations which advocate drug regimens for all HIV-positive people.

One group that stands in stark contrast is ACT UP San Francisco. David Pasquarelli its most vocal member cautions of "Deaths from strokes, heart attacks, and kidney failure" and adds: "We have lost half a dozen clients from sudden deaths in the past year and at least 30 people that have distended bellies and hunchbacks from taking the drugs".

Pasquarelli's group recently unearthed a 1997 study by San Francisco Health Department director Mitch Katz which exposes a shocking statistic which would appear to dispel the claim that the cocktails have caused AIDS deaths to plummet. Using stored blood samples and computer analyses, the study, published in the Journal of AIDS and Human Retrovirology, concluded that new HIV antibody-positive diagnoses peaked in 1982 in San Francisco-two years before HIV even had a name.

"There's a big problem in terms of looking at this as a contagious epidemic", says Pasquarelli. "HIV positive diagnoses for the past 13 years here have remained steady at 500 cases a year. People don't look at the chronology of this, or at the statistics. **They just have it in their heads that these drugs save lives, and that's it".** (Katz has since confirmed that the group interpreted his data correctly). And, Pasquarelli points out, on a national level, AIDS deaths began dropping at the end of 1994, at least three years before the drugs hit the market, a fact no one disputes.

"It is my experience that those who do not take any of these AIDS drugs are the ones who remain healthy and survive", says German physician Claus Koehnlein, who recently testified this past December at the trial of a Montreal woman who refused to give her HIV+ children cocktail therapy, and then in a chilling Orwellian scenario, had them taken from her and placed in a foster home where they are being forced to take the drugs.

"I treat the individual symptoms-the whole person, not just the virus. I treat them for whatever they are suffering from, and that's that. I have not lost a single patient in seven years and I've never used cocktail therapy". As Koehnlein wryly commented, "If you treat completely healthy people you can claim great therapeutic success".

"The vast majority - about 75 percent - of people who go on these drugs are completely healthy", says Dr. Steven Miles, AIDS researcher and doctor at UCLA Medical Center. "Large numbers of people are being inappropriately treated with drugs they don't need. And their lives are being shortened".

At Lemuel Shattuck Hospital, Massachusetts, a review was done on every HIV-positive patient who died at the hospital between May 1998 and April 1999, and compared to a group of patients who died in 1991, before drug cocktails were available. Of the 22 'post-cocktail' deaths, half died of liver toxicity from the drugs, and two more had liver toxicity listed as a secondary cause. The study concluded that liver toxicity was "now the leading cause of death among HIV-positive patients at our institution". In other words, allegedly life-saving AIDS drugs are killing AIDS patients.

Hospitals around the country are reporting radical increases in heart attacks, strokes, diabetes and other complications caused primarily by the drug's interference with the body's natural ability to metabolize fat. This is also causing the fat redistribution that leads to humpbacks and huge torsos in men, and gigantic breasts in women. At the same time, fat disappears from the face, arms and legs, rendering patients stick-like.

Holly Melroe, a Nurse at Regions Hospital in St. Paul, Minnesota, wrote last year in the Journal of the Association of Nurses in AIDS Care that the drug therapies "may have a greater life-threatening potential than the disease itself". I spoke to Melroe to see if she would confirm that statement. "Oh definitely", she said. "We are hospitalizing more people now for the side effects of the drugs, than we are for the infections of AIDS. It's a very complicated situation".

Up to 80 percent of those patients were found to have dangerously high cholesterol levels, which have led to heart attacks in many cases. One person told me he feels like his intestines are corroding from the inside out. These people can't stomach anything. They can't digest anything. They have internal organ failures. You hear stories of people who are on their way to work and they just drop dead from a heart attack. "We are seeing people who have massive swelling in the face to the point that their eyes, if they are able to open them, are incredibly sunken. The cheeks and the forehead are pushed forward. They have these hard, bumpy calcium deposits. People are bruised, almost raccoon-like around the eyes. They look like walking skulls".

Shawn O'Hearn tested positive for HIV two years ago. He, too, went on a three-drug cocktail regimen. "I was trying to be a good little boy and make it through and stay on my regimen. I was taking almost 30 pills a day". Soon his body was covered in blisters, and he was suffering debilitating nausea. He quit the drugs after four weeks, and his health returned.

The new drugs, unlike the prior generation AZT, DDI and D_4T, are very specific in their ability to inhibit HIV's crucial protease. DNA and protein are the basics of life. Protease are what control the proteins, turn them on and off, process them and so forth.

The turning point for the new drugs came in 1995, when Ho and another scientist, Dr. George Shaw, co-authored a paper, published in the scientific journal Nature, in which he detailed his new vision of HIV, AIDS and the immune system. On the day the paper was published, a press conference was held. The 'new model' was coupled with the new drugs, and a new technology took center stage - so-called viral load testing. Rather than focus on physical symptoms, the new craze was to take the drugs and measure your viral load (the amount of virus in the blood) and CD_4 cells, now considered a barometer for the immune system's health. The new drug regimens were supposed to lower the former and raise the latter. The concept was: beat back the bad guys (HIV-infected cells) and the good guys (CD_4 cells) will win.

The central puzzle of HIV research until that point had been how the HIV virus could cause AIDS, when it infected only a trivial number of T-cells - the cells AIDS patients were deficient in. As one researcher said, it was a crime scene with many more bodies than bullets.

One leading virologist who had won tremendous acclaim for having mapped the genetic structure of retroviruses and been nominated for the Nobel Prize, Dr. Peter Duesberg of the University of California-Berkeley, was sufficiently troubled by this paradox of cell infection. He concluded HIV could not be the cause of AIDS. For his heretical questioning of the AIDS establishment, he was condemned, censored in the scientific literature, no longer funded, and sent into virtual scientific exile.

Ho is not a mathematician, but nevertheless he contrived a mathematical model, on which he would base his entire premise. The model was supposed to demonstrate that HIV killed healthy cells slightly faster than they were able to replenish themselves, but the math was so dubious that very few AIDS researchers could grasp it enough to either validate or reject it. Nobody bothered to try. Instead, it simply floated upward like a balloon of epiphany, the dawn of a new era.

Now drug companies could sell drugs like never before. Consequently the lie "Miss one pill and HIV will mutate" had to be kept alive.

It was at an AIDS science conference in Florida in the early 90s that Ho, then a virologist of no particular distinction at UCLA, heard a high-ranking chemist at Abbott Pharmaceuticals discuss protease inhibitor prototypes.

Ho approached the chemist, Dale Kempf, on an airport check-in line, and told him he had a theory about "how the AIDS virus worked" and how much more ferocious it was than anybody realized. "Dale agreed that maybe we could help each other", Ho later told the Wall Street Journal.

By 1993, Abbott had narrowed its hundreds of prospective compounds down to one, which later became the most toxic of the licensed protease inhibitors, Norvir.

Meanwhile, philanthropist widow Irene Diamond had fulfilled her late husband Aaron Diamond's wish to set up a lavish research lab which would attract some of the best scientists in the country. She chose the quiet, diminutive David Ho to be the director of the institute. Ho and his colleagues began experimenting with a few patients. They gave them the cocktail therapy, measured their drug-resistant mutations, and then calculated "how many virus particles were churned out each day by infected cells". These calculations led to the infamous and *per se* deeply problematic math model.

Says Harvey Bialy, editor-at-large of the journal Nature Biotechnology: "Despite all the noise about massive viremia [levels of virus] and math models coming in from David Ho, the figures remain precisely as Peter Duesberg published in 1987 when he first critiqued the hypothesis". He adds: "Only one in 100 T-cells are ever infected, only one in 1,000 are ever making viral proteins, and that corresponds to a tiny amount of virus present in the blood. Everything else is effectively neutralized by the immune system".

"A viral load of 100,000 corresponds to one or less virus particles, which is the only medically relevant barometer. That is not enough to do anything. In the Nature paper, Ho manipulated the picture by using PCR [a technique that massively amplifies DNA] and passed it off as infectious virus. When I read it, I said, "This is f---ing nonsense! How do you pass off a biochemical unit as an infectious particle? This will never fly. But it flew".

Dr. David Rasnick, a chemist who once worked in diagnostics at Abbott and is an expert on protease inhibitors, concurs with this view. "Viral load is the most powerful microscope ever developed", he says. "If the only way you can see something is by using the most powerful microscope, how clinically relevant can it be? If a person had real viremia you wouldn't need PCR to see it. Here you're talking about a level of about one virus particle in a drop of blood!"

"Here is an example. When they look for HIV in breast milk, they do 45 cycles of PCR, which is a 35-trillion-fold amplification, in order to find enough genetic material. We are at the level of sensitivity of nuclear physics now with this PCR stuff. And David Ho talks about making HIV 'undetectable?' It starts out undetectable. That's the whole point. HIV has always been more or less undetectable".

"So they've taken a number that is next to nothing, and mass multiplied it. But it's still next to nothing. Just a bunch of numbers that are used to scare people and make people go on these drugs. All this stuff about wanting to get to zero, or to undetectable, is absurd because it implies that a single particle of HIV is lethal, but it's not" sums up Dr. Rasnick.

In the summer of 1996, thousands listened to Ho's findings from TV monitors hanging through the vast conference halls at the International AIDS Conference in Vancouver. The audience listened with rapt attention as Ho revealed his data: nine patients, he said, who had been on a combination of drugs including some of the new protease inhibitors, had "no evidence of the virus in their bloodstream", after being on the drugs for between 90 and 300 days. Ho calmly repeated his mantra: because of the new drugs, it was "time to hit HIV, early and hard".

"It was just unadulterated hype. It was preposterous", recalls Dr. Steven Miles. "It was almost like an instantaneous religion, or a cult, right after Vancouver. You were either a part of that hit-hard-hit-early religion or you were not. It split the HIV community".

AIDS treatment was in a depressed state at this time. The results of a devastating study three years earlier had dashed the long-held belief that AZT could extend life - instead, it was shown to shorten life. Many prominent researchers, deeply alarmed that they had unconsciously given a drug that had done more harm than good, were abandoning toxic drugs and looking to resolve the disease by stimulating the immune system instead. But Ho's mathematical model which 'demonstrated' that the virus was 'furiously replicating', made the virus suddenly seem more lethal than ever, and in the fervor that followed, doctors who advocated being careful and conservative with drug regimens were seen as foolish pacifists, willfully surrendering to a vicious enemy. A kind of collective fantasy formed in the hushed room at the Vancouver conference, as the low-key scientist unveiled his data, never altering his blank facial expression, but inspiring a mania with his quiet use of a few new buzzwords: 'eradication', 'undetectable'. The fantasy was that the new drugs could eradicate HIV - get rid of it - and that once it was gone, people could stop taking the drugs and live AIDS-free for the rest of their lives. All agreed that these drugs were not designed for long term use, that they were way too toxic.

Ho cast a powerful spell over not just his audience, but the world's media, medical community, and AIDS community. The excitement that emanated from Ho's presentation was palpable - it spread like wildfire through the media. Within hours, people were rushing in to their doctors' offices, begging for prescriptions. Most of them were healthy. None of them cared about anything except the new magic word: eradication.

"It is not even really a mathematical model", says Mark Craddock, a mathematician at the University of Technology-Sydney, referring to Ho's construct. "In my opinion, it's mathematical junk". Craddock has written several critiques of Ho's model, and says he cannot comprehend how it was ever able to gain such momentum. "Ho's equations predict that over the course of 10 years, an HIV-positive person will produce more particles of HIV than there are atoms in the universe. There is no way you could make that much virus".

An editorial in the February 1998 issue of Nature Medicine by renowned virologist Mario Roederer pointed out that cocktail therapy does not cause T-cells to increase, but rather to be redistributed throughout the body - which is not an immunological advantage. This had been discovered a year earlier when an American group of researchers developed a way to 'tag' newly synthesized DNA and isolate T-cell populations. What they found does not bode well for those who are on cocktail drugs: of three groups – uninfected people, untreated HIV-positive people, and HIV-positive people on the drugs - the T-cells of the ones on the drugs survived the shortest amount of time.

"You don't have to waste a lot of time on this", says Bialy when I ask him about how and when Ho's research was refuted in the scientific literature. "The Roederer piece finished it. Ho is finished. In the scientific world right now it is firmly established that the model is nonsense".

Veteran AIDS doctor Joseph Sonnabend, co-founder of AmFAR, scowls when I ask about Ho's math model. "Of course it's wrong", he says impatiently. "Everybody knows that. It's such way-out bullshit. The RNA of retroviruses turns into DNA and becomes part of us. It's part of our being. You can't ever get rid of it".

Ho had committed spurious research by withholding a vital finding from the data. In his experiments, Ho had shown that protease inhibitors, by stopping HIV allowed healthy CD_4 cells to flourish. But what he didn't reveal was that CD_8 cells (which have nothing to do with HIV) also increased.

"I heard from a well-placed source that protease inhibitors were approved by the FDA, based on Ho's Nature paper", says David Rasnick. "There was certainly no clinical data that they were effective, and to this day there is still none". The rush to get the new AIDS drugs on the market caused a near-total disintegration of the FDA drug approval process. Some of these drugs were approved in a matter of weeks, a process that normally takes years. Protease inhibitors were approved on small, short trials, in which results were virtually engineered. Data can be skewed to show anything under such circumstances. Some - especially AIDS - drugs these days are tested in the human population - after they are released.

Towards the end of 1997, a study from Germany showed that almost half of those taking protease inhibitors had their virus levels increase, not decrease. The authors wrote: "The success seen in controlled studies is not necessarily reflected in everyday practice".

A few years before protease inhibitors came onto the market, Rasnick attended a conference where a paper authored by Dr. Paul Saftig, and published in the journal EMBO, was presented. It had no relationship to AIDS, but nonetheless stayed vivid in his memory.

It was a so-called 'knock-out' experiment, in which scientists totally erase a gene from an animal, and then gauge what effect it has. The gene is erased from either a fertilized or non-fertilized egg then implanted, and then the resulting offspring, if there are any, are studied. "Typically what happens", says Rasnick, "is that either the animals are born with absolutely no difference that you detect, or you don't get any offspring at all".

But this experiment was highly unusual. In it, scientists removed an aspartyl protease known as cathepsin D - one that all humans have - from the mice. The mice were all born normal, and for the first three weeks of their lives, appeared to be thriving. But on the 21st day, every last one of them died. Autopsies showed that the mice had starved to death. "Their intestines were completely destroyed", says Rasnick. "Also, they had what the authors called fulminate loss of T-cells and B-cells. In other words, their immune systems were shot".

"That study was a real red flag", says Rasnick. "Cathepsin D is the only protease I know that is absolutely essential for life, so you'd want to stay away from it. I remember thinking to myself at the time, thank God we are not working on aspartyl proteases, or making inhibitors for them".

When Rasnick began hearing stories of the chronic diarrhea and wasting syndrome that was among many problems to afflict people on the new protease inhibitors, he had a sinking feeling. "I said, 'Oh shit, it's happening'. You see, there's always crossover. Even though it's not the target, all of these protease inhibitors also inhibit cathepsin D. The same aspartyl protease that they knocked out in the mice".

"And they're giving people up to seven grams a day of this stuff. I don't see how anybody can survive that in the long run. I'd love to see some post-mortems done on these guys who die on cocktails. I'd like to see what their intestines look like". Rasnick believes it was a grave mistake for the FDA ever to approve protease inhibitors for human use. "I would pull these protease inhibitors off the market based on the Saftig paper alone".

In March of last year, a gathering of the world's leading AIDS researchers was convened, as they do each year, at the elite Chemotherapy of AIDS Conference, known as the Gordon Conference, in Ventura, California. Nearly half of the 105 people attending were from within the pharmaceutical industry. David Ho was there, as was Martin Markowitz. Markowitz and Ho received a lot of publicity for their ongoing study of 27 people on HAART (Highly Active Anti-retroviral Therapy) - the multidrug regimen that is now the standard of care for AIDS patients, both adults and children - in fact, even pregnant women.

"At last year's conference, I asked Markowitz if his patients on HAART were doing better, the same, or worse while on the drugs", says Dr. Rasnick. "He didn't say a word. He just stood there. I asked the question three times. This time I decided not to ask. If his patients had been doing well, I'm sure he would have let us all know, especially me".

Dr. William Cameron, consultant to the Canadian FDA, "completely demolished the viral load surrogate marker" as a relevant way to measure health or the success of treatments, according to Rasnick. He used as an example the clinical disaster, never reported in the media, of a drug many people were on years ago called DDI. Over a 12-week study, the drug worked brilliantly on viral load levels, but shortly thereafter turned out to be virulently toxic, in fact lethally so. At the highly private conference, where no press is allowed and attendees are told not to discuss what they hear, even Ho recanted his central tenant, and said, "Viremia [viral levels] are not predictive of clinical outcome". Adds Rasnick: "These guys will admit this between themselves, they just don't admit it publicly".

The AIDS magazine POZ and others like it are filled with protease inhibitor ads that drastically contrast with the cruel reality. The ads feature muscular, tanned, and beautiful people at the peak of their powers: climbing mountains, sprinting over hurdles, sailing, and generally beaming with life. In reality, three years into the protease inhibitor craze, most people on cocktail therapy can barely function. I talked to one of the most well-known protease models, Michael Weathers, whose handsome face adorns several billboards across America, and he said that he had not only never taken protease inhibitors, but had never taken any AIDS drugs. He is perfectly healthy 13 years after learning he was positive. "They have this rule that they have to use HIV-positive models for their AIDS drug ads", Weathers comments, "but they certainly do not use models who are using their drugs. That would hardly make for effective advertising".

The list of side effects listed by the drug companies themselves in their own ads is so long, it numbers in the hundreds. The toxic effects are so numerous, they have broken them down into categories. Within each of those body systems, up to 50 specific symptoms are listed. For one of the drugs, Saquinavir, under 'Adverse reactions', are listed : 'intracranial hemorrhage leading to death' and 'pancreatitis leading to death'.

Leafing through POZ, I read the fine print that follows every protease ad. In each and every one, it states that the drugs have killed people. Yet the accompanying text warns about the importance of staying on the drugs no matter what. Be smart, one ad for the Glaxo drug Combivir advises: Without your HIV drugs, there's nothing to stop the virus from making billions of copies of itself. Next time you're tempted to skip a dose or two, think again. HIV drugs should be taken on time, every day. That's the only way known to keep enough of each drug in your blood at all times to fight HIV.

I set off in search of ground zero, a beginning, a place where the tornado started turning. I call people who work on the inside of the AIDS machine. They all speak - angrily, but fearfully - of a pharmaceutical industry that makes its presence felt to reporters, scientists, doctors, and AIDS activists. As Dr. Sonnabend put it, "The drug companies are present in some way in virtually every single moment of my professional career".

"It is absolutely extraordinary", says Dr. Miles, who says he has been on various drug companies blacklists for saying negative things about their products. "People don't realize all the myriad ways that doctors benefit from the drug companies. For example, let's say that drug company 'A' likes the message that Dr. C is talking about. They give a research grant to Dr. C and because it's listed as a 'research grant', people will say, 'Oh well, this is above board', when in fact it's nothing more than a glorified under-the-table payment. Miles adds "Now, let's say that you are Dr. C, and you have a $250,000 research grant from company 'A'. What is the likelihood that you are going to say anything bad about their drugs? Zero. At best you are going to say nothing". Miles has felt the heat of this situation personally, being one of the few mainstream AIDS doctors who stood up and resisted the hit-hard-hit-early mania.

"Just go to the U.S. Public Health Service web site. Under federal law they have to disclose whom they have taken money from. Some of these doctors have taken money from 15 to 20 different companies. If 20 companies that are in the business of making money for drug treatments are giving you money can you honestly stand up and say, don't treat!"

Another man, who for years has worked on the inside of AIDS research, implores me not to print his name, swearing he will be out of a job immediately if I do. "Look at the media, that's where it happens", he said. "Look at those earliest pieces about Ho and the cocktails that ran in the Wall Street Journal. They are just pure propaganda, pure drug company puff pieces. And those reporters won the Pulitzer that year for their AIDS reporting. The pharmaceutical industry exerts a huge influence on scientists and journalists".

"You have to understand that these AIDS journalists have very close relationships with the drug companies, with their PR people. That affects how things get reported. I mean, they fund everything. They fund all the research, first of all. There is almost no such thing as independent research. All clinical trials are paid for by the drug companies". He laughs when I express alarm at this. "My God are you naive! Everybody - not just David Ho - the reporters, the doctors, everybody is part of this system. They're all part of the same club, and they all play the same game. They all have the same, big egos. And nobody - certainly not the reporters - is going to stand up and wave their finger and say, 'This is all a big horrible machine!' You know why? Because they're all profiting from it.

Dr. Leo Rebello's Note : After reading this Damning Verdict on pharmaceutical mafia's mediocre agent David Ho, what say you on protease inhibitors? Aids Patients, stand up and fight for your fundamental right to refuse poisons. Right to Choose, Right to Health, Right to Life are the most fundamental of all human rights, among other rights that civilized societies enjoy.

DR. LEO REBELLO'S REPORT ON XIII INTERNATIONAL AIDS CONFERENCE, DURBAN, SOUTH AFRICA.

1. At the XIII International AIDS Conference, 9th to 15th July, 2000 (Durban, South Africa), I presented a 6 hours workshop on AIDS AND HOLISTIC HEALING at which Indian Ambassador and Indian Minister of Health, among others, were present. Christine Maggiore (popular author of "What if everyuthing you thought you knew about AIDS WAS WRONG?") along with her film-maker husband, child and mother attended it and also received healing. The manual on AIDS and Holistic Healing, written by me, and which was published by the Conference organizers for distribution among the participants, ran short because of more-than-expected response to my workshop.
2. Participated in a Satellite Conference by India Caucus and spoke on "From AIDS SCARE to AIDS CARE".
3. Guided the African Traditional Healers in their day long deliberations.
4. Participated in half a day panel discussion on Alternative Medicine at UNISA.
5. Helped organise and led a historic World Traditional Healers March which was reported widely both by electronic and print media.
6. Participated in the Breakfast meeting organised by the Indian High Commissioner in SA at which some 200 Indian delegates, MPs, Indian Minister of Health, two other State Ministers were present.

7. Participated in the Mayor's cocktails and dinner meeting. Since I am a teetotaler, I had only fruit cocktails!

8. Had a meeting with the Conference Chair, Dr. Jerry Coovadia.

9. Participated with the Ugandan Ambassadors of Hope in their deliberation on how religion can be used for dissemination of HIV/AIDS and family norms information.

10. My poem AIDS NO MORE was used at a public function on 8th July where the Mayor of Durban and African Minister of Social Welfare, among others, were present.

11. I was interviewed by the Radio, Press and Television. SABC showed the Traditional Healers March and my interview several times and photographs appeared in several papers.

12. Participated in Poetry Reading session at a Museum complex. Enroute to the venue lost way and I hailed six pillion-riding policemen, who kindly offered to drop me at the venue. While I read about foreigners being mugged in Durban / Johannesburg, I merged with the locals very well. Many people even spoke to me in their local lingo and I had to tell them that I was from Bombay and had come here for AIDS conference.

13. After the AIDS Conference, participated in another four days International Conference on Non Violence.

14. My poem titled SHARING as also speech at the said Peace Conference were much appreciated.

15. Ms Ela Gandhi, MP, grand daughter of Mahatma Gandhi, who facilitated my participation in the International Conference on Non-Violence, also took me to show her grandfather's work in Phoenix settlements, which she is carrying on.

After the two conferences, I went to Shakhaland (Zulu Land), Pretoria, Witbank (to treat AIDS patients), Johannesburg, Cape Town, Cape End and the Robben Island (where Nelson Mandela was incarcerated for 18 out of 27 years of jail term)

On my return journey I took a halt in Mauritius for four days and lectured there too.

MEET ON AIDS & AM

In the second week of November 2000, WHO, UNAIDS, ICMR, Indian Government's Department of Indian Systems of Medicine and others took a step towards giving a seal of scientific approval and credibility to Alternative Medicines for AIDS. At the said meet in Delhi (to which I was invited, but could not go due to prior commitments), it was reported that Ayurvedic, Siddha and Homeopathy research in HIV/AIDS was being carried out at the following centres in India :

At the Central Council for Research in Homeopathy in Delhi, Mumbai and Chennai, since 1992. At Tilak Ayurveda Mahavidyala and Hospital, Pune, Maharashtra, since 1995. At the Ayurvedic Wing of Amala Cancer Hospital, Thrissur, Kerala, since 1995. At Hospital for Thoracic and Chest Medicine, Tambaram, Tamil Nadu, since 1998. At Jamnagar and Surat Medical Colleges, supported by Gujarat Government, since the beginning of 2000.

It was in 1976, the World Health Assembly acknowledged the potential value of traditional medicine in expanding health services by calling attention to the manpower reserve constituted by traditional health practitioners (resolution WHA29.72).

In the following year, another resolution (WHA30.49) urged countries to utilize their traditional systems of medicine. Yet another resolution was passed in 1978, in which WHO was called upon to develop a comprehensive approach to the subject of medicinal plants (WHA31.33). Nine years later, in 1987, the Fortieth World Health Assembly reaffirmed the main points of the earlier resolutions, as well as related recommendations made at the International Conference on Primary Health Care, held in Alma-Ata, USSR, in 1978 (WHA40.33). In 1989, a resolution was passed (WHA42.43) that recalled earlier resolutions on traditional medicine, traditional health practitioners, and traditional remedies and affirmed that together they constitute a comprehensive approach to the utilization of medicinal plants in the health services. **Why was this not taken up for so long?**

STATEMENT OF DR. LEO REBELLO
ISSUED ON THE OCCASION OF UNGASS (25-27 June, 2001)
Circulated worldwide and published on several websites.

Crows, like cockroaches, are ubiquitous wherever there is garbage. Since I have not visited USA, I would not know whether they have crows and cockroaches there. But from June 25, to participate in UNGASS, "crows from all countries" will assemble in New York and their 'caw-caw' will be so deafening that any logical thinking, that after 20 years AIDS has not spread into the general population as predicted, will be drowned. Every one will return after a brief, all-expenses-paid holiday, and the following facts will be lost sight of:

1. That the disturbing numbers of global AIDS cases touted by UNAIDS are based on 'guesstimates'. The commonly cited figure of 55 million AIDS victims worldwide is a projection that contrasts starkly with the WHO's total of 2.3 million global AIDS cases in 20 years.

2. That 90% of AIDS cases in USA are found in two official risk groups, Men Having Sex with Men (MSM) and Injection Drug Users (IDU), and that over 80% of AIDS diagnosed are males.

3. That despite paranoid estimates of 4 to 5 million HIV/AIDS cases in S.Africa, less than 15,000 actual cases of AIDS have been counted in South Africa in the past two decades.

4. That the toxic effects of ARVs include nerve damage, weakened bones, unusual accumulation of fat in the neck and abdomen and drug-induced diabetes. Many people have developed dangerously high levels of cholesterol and other lipids in the blood, raising concern that HIV positive persons might face another epidemic of heart diseases and cancers.

5. That AIDS is the consequence of a suppressed immune system which has been subjected to repeated onslaughts by four factors that build up toxins and deficiencies in the body. These are: antibiotic abuse, recreational drug abuse, anal sex (which causes toxic shock to the receiving partner) and nutritional stress.

6. That the damage caused by the stressed immune system could be reversed by good diet, yogic and other exercises, herbs available readily, acupuncture, homeopathy, proper rest, avoidance of alcohol, drugs, tobacco, proper hygiene, etc. In other words, a person is to be treated as a whole : body, mind and spirit.

And so many other factors that militate for attention. I wonder what the investigative press of America, which brought out Watergate and forced Richard Nixon to resign, is doing. Or for that matter what is the International Press doing? Why is it sleeping? Have the pharmaceutical MNCs given it some sleeping pills?

Finally, if tobacco giant Philip Morris could be ordered to cough up $3 bn as damages to a smoker for purposely lying/deceiving by hiding the fact that smoking is addictive and causes lung cancer and other diseases; why, oh why all those MNCs which make money by selling lethal drugs to AIDS victims, by hiding in small prints the facts that these drugs are not life saving, but life threatening, cannot be sued? At least smoking is voluntary. ARVs are compulsorily prescribed to unsuspecting patients. Do you people know that Prescription Addiction and Aids by Prescription pose a greater threat to humanity than deadly Arms and Mines?

DR. LEO REBELLO'S REPORT ON XIV INTERNATIONAL AIDS CONFERENCE HELD IN BARCELONA, SPAIN

The 14th International AIDS Conference, held in Barcelona, Spain, (from 6th to 12 July, 2002) was nothing but a circus - with 17,000 participants, leaders like Bill Clinton, IK Gujral baffing, Health Minister of India Shatrughan Sinha reading from the notes passed by mediocre Secretaries, Bachi Karkaria-type journalists asking foolish questions to mark their presence, practically 90% delegates smoking and freaking out, after collecting their *per diem* (210 Euros each, in addition to free air ticket, free accommodation, free transport, free food and gifts), Barcelona turned out into the biggest tourist destination. I was the ONLY stupid person who did not take one day, half-day, two-days sightseeing tours.

The "official" conference dealt with anti-retrovirals, anti-retrovirals, and anti-retrovirals ! Nothing on Alternative Medicine, Alternative Methods, Alternative Approaches. Durban AIDS Conference 2000 was decidedly much better in every respect. The next jamboree is in Thailand in 2004.

If only I had collected the papers/things strewn everywhere on the last day at the Conference venue in Barcelona, and transported to India, I would make atleast two million rupees by selling that waste! What a criminal waste of resources. One glaring example should suffice : Glaxo gave to each and every delegate bags, pens, medals, CDs, coffee flasks, mugs, books, posters and unlimited flow of coffee and tea, not to speak of luncheons and parties, because it has made the biggest profits by selling anti-retrovirals, ostensibly by saving the poor AIDS patients dying in Africa, Asia and Latin America !

The parallel AIDS conference which did NOT believe in HIV = AIDS = DEATH paradigm, at which I was one of the main speakers along with Roberto Giraldo, Etienne de Harven, was more challenging. But since it was NOT sponsored, it lacked in funds, and consequently there were about 500 participants as against 17,000 participants at the "official" conference. But it was well covered by the media.

On my return journey, I spent one day in Paris, and then three days each in Kuwait and Dubai, lecturing Indians, who liked my lectures and healing methods so much, that they have decided to host me again.

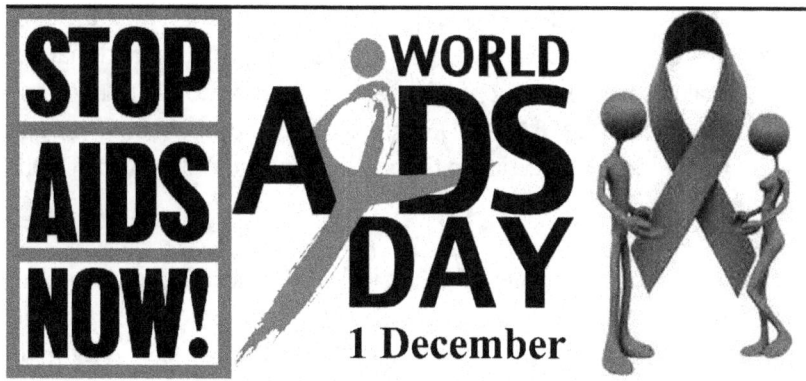

SUMMARY OF THE INTERNATIONAL MEETING FOR THE SCIENTIFIC REAPPRASING OF AIDS
Barcelona, July 8-11, 2002

Report prepared by:
Roberto Giraldo, MD, United States (RobGiraldo@aol.com),
Alfredo Embid, acupuncturist & writer, Spain (amcmh@amcmh.org),
Delia Arellano, journalist, Mexico (deliaaarellano@yahoo.com.mx),
Ángel Galeano, writer, Colombia (arteyciencia2001@hotmail.com) and
Leo Rebello, N.D., Ph.D., D.Sc., India (leorebello@vsnl.com)

While agencies of the government of the United States (CDC, NIH, DHHS), pharmaceutical corporations, WHO, and the Population Council were meeting at the Palau St. Jordi in Barcelona at their "XIV World Conference on HIV/AIDS", continuing their deceptions of all the world's people, a group of so-called "AIDS dissidents" were meeting at La Farinera del Clot, a culture and arts center of the Barcelona Municipality, in an "International Meeting for the Scientific Reappraising of AIDS", organized by the Spanish National Association of Complementary Medicines (AMC). About 500 people attended from Spain, Portugal, France, Germany, Italy, England, Ireland, Mexico, Colombia, India, Cameroon, and the United States, including daily participants.

Monday July 8
1. <u>OPENING.</u> Mrs. Ruse Veciana, of the Human Rights Counsel of Barcelona City Hall, gave the opening address. She explained that her presence at this meeting honored the right of all people to information and to understand all sides of the AIDS controversy. She promised to present the conclusions of this meeting to the government authorities of Barcelona and Spain.

2. Some historic issues of the AIDS dissident movement: Roberto Giraldo, MD, from the United States, briefly explained the main scientific arguments against the widely accepted belief that HIV is the cause of AIDS. He described the basics of the scientific proposal that AIDS is a toxic and nutritional syndrome caused by the alarming worldwide increment of immunological stressor agents (oxidizing agents). He explained briefly the non-toxic alternatives for the prevention and treatment of AIDS. He pointed out the major contributions of Peter Duesberg, from Berkeley, California, and Eleni Papadopulos-Eleopulos, from the Australian Perth Group.

Joan Shenton, from England (meditel@joanshenton.clara.co.uk), explained the sharp difficulties that she encountered trying to document the dissident hypothesis, from her first videos to her book Positively False.

Alfredo Embid, from Spain, presented a critical description of the supporters of the official Conference; the CDC, NIH, WHO, the Population Council, etc.

3. Living witnesses. A dozen 'seropositive' people and people diagnosed with AIDS, from several countries described their personal histories. Many of them were addicted to recreational drugs in the past. None of them are currently using orthodox treatments. All have a normal life, avoiding as much as possible exposures to toxic substances. All use a variety of natural measures to detoxify and stimulate weakened cells, tissues and systems. All are healthy and full of energy.

4. Opening of an exhibit of photographs, Our Endangered Species, by Diana Giraldo, from the United States (dg718ny@aol.com). Comprising 80 photographs, the exhibit documents the diversity of toxic agents that have markedly increased worldwide and that are the actual cause of both the general deterioration of health and of particular immune deficiencies.

5. Presentation of the video Looking for Solutions, by Joan Shenton, from England (meditel@joanshenton.clara.co.uk). The video includes an interview with President Thabo Mbeki of South Africa. The audience heard the South African President's points of view regarding AIDS.

President Mbeki described in detail the widespread censorship of alternative views regarding AIDS and insisted that Africa's priority must be to relieve poverty and its consequences. Although the video had been aired in several African countries, this was its European premier.

Tuesday July 9
LECTURES ON THE CONTROVERSY ABOUT THE CAUSES AND SOLUTIONS FOR AIDS

1. Immunological Stressor Agents are the Real Cause of AIDS, by Roberto Giraldo, MD, from the United States. This lecture was presented in honor of the memory of Huw Christie, Editor and Manager of Continuum magazine. Giraldo explained the epidemiological, biologic, and common sense reasons for believing that what is known as HIV is not the cause of AIDS. He described the scientific bases for AIDS being the maximum state of deterioration that a person can suffer as a consequence of involuntary, sometimes voluntary, multiple, repeated, and chronic exposures to stressor agents (oxidizing agents) that are significantly increasing worldwide. These agents can have a chemical, physical, biological, mental, or nutritional (lack of food in underdeveloped countries and excess of junk food in developed countries) origin. He explained the scientific bases for effective and non-toxic alternatives for the treatment and prevention of AIDS as a toxic and nutritional syndrome.

2. HIV Has Never Been Isolated, by Etienne de Harven, MD, from France (pitou.deharven@wanadoo.fr). Numerous scientific reasons were presented for believing that neither Luc Montagnier, nor Robert Gallo, nor Jay Levy ever isolated the virus that came to be called HIV. Attendees were delighted by the manner in which de Harven detailed the technical reasons behind the absence of an electron microscopy photograph of what is known as the AIDS virus. He explained that in 1997 two groups of researchers in the United States, France, and Germany again failed to isolate HIV, even though this time they followed the established steps for the isolation of retroviruses. He explained that if HIV did indeed exist it would be straightforward to isolate it from individuals having high viral load counts. In this regard, he has proposed this very experiment and it will be carried out as one of the experiments proposed by the dissidents at the South African Presidential AIDS Advisory Panel.

3. Other Causes of Immune Deficiency, by Alfredo Embid, from Spain. Examples of a wide variety of chemical, physical, biological, mental, and nutritional agents that cause immune deficiency were presented. The examples included medications like antiretrovirals, pesticides like Aldicarb, and industrial pollutants like dioxines. Embid pointed out that responsibility for these agents fell on the companies that manufacture them and explained that some of these same companies are sponsors of the official World Conferences on HIV/AIDS. He described in detail the growing problem of ionizing radiation, due to the growth of the industrial/military complex since 1945 and to the bombings carried out by the United States and its allies on several countries with weapons said to contain no uranium. He explained the different degenerative diseases that are being caused by radiation worldwide.

4. Psychosocial Implications of AIDS, Tom DiFerdinando, from the United States (DaleRiever@aol.com). Using philosophical explanations, the official view of AIDS as an infectious, viral, and contagious illness was characterized as blaming and isolating 'seropositive' individuals, people with AIDS, and everyone else. There is a growing spiritual isolation among people and between people and all natural beings. DiFerdinando pointed out that the orthodox view of AIDS exacerbates this spiritual isolation. Today, not many care about fellowbeings or about nature. We must return to a spirit of solidarity and love, and respect ourselves, our fellow human beings, and all other inhabitants of the universe.

5. The Chaotic Consequences of the Myth about the Transmission of AIDS, Roberto Giraldo, MD, from the United States. Giraldo described references in the medical literature from June 1981 through April 1984, before the phenomenon known as HIV came onto the stage. These references demonstrate that the CDC, together with other agencies of the United States government and the World Health Organization, unleashed upon the world a rumor about the transmission of AIDS, a rumor having no scientific basis. This rumor evolved into a myth. He described in detail the terrible consequences of this myth for male homosexuals, for hemophiliacs, for people of both genders in the underdeveloped countries of Africa and other continents, for health care workers, and for everyone else.

6. Retroviruses and Cancer, of Rats and Men, Etienne de Harven, MD, from France. Prof. Harven witnessed the research done during the 70's and 80's attempting to assign viruses-specifically, retroviruses-as the cause of cancer. He described the multimillion dollar sums spent on frustrating investigations which were unable to demonstrate the initial hypothesis. When AIDS started at the beginning of the 80's, it came like "a ring to a finger" to the frustrated researchers of the "war on cancer" program of the United States government. He explained how the institutions for cancer research became institutions for AIDS research and how the frustrated cancer researchers became AIDS researchers, transferring to AIDS science the idea of viruses as a cause.

7. The Causes of AIDS in Africa, Roberto Giraldo, MD, from the United States. Giraldo noted that one of the ways to determine whether or not AIDS exists in Africa is through the careful study of publications that describe patients with AIDS from African countries before 1984, when HIV came onto the stage and "infected" AIDS research. He described other facts that favor the existence of AIDS in Africa: changes in the behavior of infectious, parasitic, degenerative and tumor diseases in recent decades in African countries; and changes in morbidity rates, mortality rates and the decrease in life span in several African countries. He described the scientific evidence demonstrating that multiple, repeated, and chronic exposures to infectious and parasitic diseases, in combination with other consequences of poverty, deteriorate the immune system as well as other body systems. He explained that the consequences of poverty are being transmitted from generation to generation in a cumulative way, and that therefore neither poverty nor malnutrition are static phenomena that have always existed in Africa, as stated by defenders of HIV. He explained that the fact that AIDS exists in Africa and that its causes are different from those in developed countries is an indicator that the human species itself is endangered. He emphasized that the official view of HIV/AIDS does not permit us to fully perceive the seriousness of the situation.

Concert by Spanish singer Mara del Alar and guitar player Álvaro Carpi (Alvaro.Carpi@uv.es). After a long day of technical, scientific, economic, and political discussions concerning the controversy about the causes of and solutions for AIDS, it was very rewarding to hear this marvelous concert featuring songs and music from different Spanish speaking countries. There will always be a place in our hearts for these two artists.

Wednesday July 10
SEMINAR ABOUT NON-TOXIC ALTERNATIVES FOR THE TREATMENT AND PREVENTION OF AIDS

1. Scientific bases for non-toxic alternatives for the treatment and prevention of AIDS. Roberto Giraldo, MD, United States.
2. Essential oils. Ferdinando Pissani, Italy (productions@mclink.it).
3. Ocean Plasma. Laureano Domínguez (laldormar@latinmail.com) & Wílmer Soler, MD (wsoler@medicina.udea.edu.co), Spain/Colombia.
4. Body Work. Tom DiFerdinando, New York (DaleRiever@aol.com).
5. Eastern Medicine. Mechanisms of action and review of experimental papers. Alfredo Embid, Spain (amcmh@amcmh.org).
6. Naturopathic Medicine and AIDS. Pedro Ródenas, MD, Spain (natura@aticaediciones.com).
7. AIDS and Traditional Medicines: Yoga, Nutrition, Homeopathic Medicine, etc. Leo Rebello, ND, Ph.D., D.Sc., India.
8. The mind, the mirror and the last herb. Fintan Dunne, Ireland (kathymcmahon@eircom.net).
9. Holotropic Breathing/Induced Vibration and other states of consciousness. Manuel Almendro, Spain (oxigeme@isid.es).

Through the entire day, lecturers from different countries described in detail the mechanisms by which a variety of non-toxic therapies are currently used, highly effectively and at very low cost, for the treatment and prevention of AIDS, for example :

10. Leo Rebello, N.D., Ph.D., D.Sc., from India, said that like there are life saving medicines, there are also live saving exercises. Yoga can halt or reverse the progression of AIDS. Quoting from his book AIDS AND ALTERNATIVE MEDICINE he said that "scientists were discovering now what folk wisdom has always known : You can worry yourself sick. You can grieve yourself to death".

"Out of this research has emerged a new branch in medicine : psycho-neuro-immunology, a blend of psychology, neurology and immunology". He emphasised that "good nutrition, proper exercise, adequate sleep, relaxation, meditation, breathing practice of paced respiration enhances the immune function. Whereas, poor diet, inactivity, insomnia, somnolence, constant stress, smoking, heavy alcohol consumption, depresses the immune function".

Dr. Leo Rebello, President, AIDS Alternativa International, cautioned the poor people of Africa that they, instead of begging for free supply of deleterious anti-retrovirals, should demand adequate fruits like jackfruit, yellow bananas, papaya, black grapes, carrot, spinach, grapefruit, lemon and radish and herbs like Echinacea, Hypericum, Garlic, Lycopus, Mango leaves, horse radish, Neem, Bear's garlic which are specific for boosting their immunity.

Rebello further said : "AIDS victims must have alkaline diet, naturally grown food with high vitamin and mineral content and low in proteins. Infact animal proteins, which are touted as very effective body builders, are the main cause of cancers and other viral load. If the body is strong, AIDS or any other virus, germ will not attack, as food builds up the regenerative forces of the body". He further emphasised that for the so-called opportunistic infections there were many safer, cheaper, more effective biochemic, homoepathic and ayurvedic medicines and also alternative vaccines and approaches. He demanded that the medical hegemony of orthodox medicine must end and WHO should implement all the resolutions of World Health Assembly which has recognised Alternative Medicines. He reiterated his demand of making available atleast 25% of research funds to Alternative Medicine. Rebello rounded up his seminar with a practical session on relaxation technique and meditation, which was appreciated by all.

11. In the audience were about one hundred alternative, complimentary or holistic therapists who have been preventing or treating AIDS with excellent results, enriching the discussions with their knowledge and expertise. Also, a group of "seropositive" individuals and some, who had AIDS in the past, described the simple ways in which they were able to prevent or overcome AIDS and the fact that they are currently enjoying healthy lives.

12. It was emphasized that it is important to continue building an international network with those institutions, health care professionals, and alternative/complimentary therapists that are currently preventing or healing AIDS without antiretroviral or any other toxic medication. It is important that they communicate among themselves, exchange knowledge and experiences, and record their techniques and results.

13. Alternative treatment of 200 HIV-positive patients from different countries: "Health is not a prescription; it is a discipline." Juan José Flores, MD, PhD, Mexico (drjuanflores@yahoo.com); Mohamed Al-Bayati, PhD, DABT, United States (maalbayati@toxi-health.com); Christine Maggiore, United States (Christine@aliveandwell.org); Alejandro Flores, United States (alex81@earthlink.net). From 1998 to 2001, 200 patients were seen in Xalapa-Veracruz, Mexico.

14. The analysis of 10 of the 200 patients reveals additional evidence that AIDS is not caused by a retrovirus named HIV, but that its development depends on multiple factors. In most patients it was easy to revert their immunological abnormalities, even those that were severe. All patients were treated in a similar way:

a) Antiretrovirals are suspended;
b) Nutritional alterations are treated by rigorous diet intervention;
c) Vitamin supplements were given;
d) Oral lipoic acid;
e) Permanent psychological help;
f) If necessary, specific treatment for infections is administered. Neither did HIV status influence decisions nor were AIDS tests ordered.

Unfortunately this research was not presented at the meeting because Dr. Flores, once in Spain, was intentionally sent to a different city.

Theatrical production by the Grupo de Teatro Atzavara from Tortosa, Spain. Performed by a solo actor criticizing the official view on HIV/AIDS. Concert by Apollinaire Dschoutezo, a songwriter and musician of African Jazz from Cameroon.

Thursday July 11
ROUND TABLE: THE MEDIA AND THE CONTROVERSY ABOUT THE CAUSES OF AND SOLUTIONS FOR AIDS

1. Guillermo Caba, journalist, Spain (gcaba@hotmail.com). "It seems that there is no solution in the way that they describe the problems today; there is a crisis of paradigms and the media, instead of promoting light, make a living by healing illnesses" … "The language used by the major media is improper, they try to complicate everything with weird words, creating a bad ambience. Popular language may help us a lot. We need to learn from those who are happy and optimistic. I believe that the way I say things is more important than the things themselves."

2. Delia Arellano, journalist, reporter of the newspaper El Bravo from Matamoros, Mexico (deliaaarellano@yahoo.com.mx). She explained how, from a case diagnosed as AIDS in a woman from Matamoros, Mexico, her coworker and photographer, Héctor Lozada, upon seeing in a newspaper a "photo of the AIDS virus," realized that the photo was not a real photograph, and started to investigate the medical records of the patient diagnosed with AIDS. He found that what she really had was tuberculosis. Her physician had not realized it and, thanks to the work of the journalist, the treatment was corrected. Since then both journalists, Delia and Héctor, have continued to report upon similar cases that were diagnosed as AIDS using non-specific tests, in different states of Mexico, but that were in reality other diseases. These two journalists have been fortunate in having the support of their managers in the newspaper El Bravo. They have published several articles containing dissident views about AIDS. The newspaper has a very large readership and there are now workers from 150 factories in the region who are interested in the subject and have contacted them. They have even been contacted by several physicians who did not know about the dissident views of AIDS. "We know that the number of AIDS cases has declined in this State" … "We came to this meeting to let you know about this modest work and to let you know that we will continue in this struggle as AIDS dissident journalists."

3. Héctor Lozada, journalist, reporter of the newspaper El Bravo from Matamoros, Mexico (fototeto@yahoo.com.mx). From his job as a reporter he knows that journalists do not have a critical spirit, most journalists do not question official views and report the things that they are told without asking for proof. "I believe many of my colleagues neither question individuals at the governmental level, nor those from large centers of research, nor those from the pharmaceutical companies. We write exactly in the way that we are told, even knowing that this or that is not true ... There is a lack of common sense in understanding subjects and problems. For example, in Luck Montagnier's book, he explains that there are people who develop AIDS who are HIV-negative, who die from AIDS. However, journalists do not care about this contradiction ... A similar thing happens with discrepancies between Gallo and Montagnier regarding the origin of AIDS, discrepancies which are published, but nobody says a word. Similarly with information from the CDC; they replied to me that viral load is improper for diagnosing HIV infection, yet nobody calls them on this, most journalists do not question it, they just report that viral load diagnoses HIV infection ... In the future, we journalists should compromise ourselves in seeking truth and should not let those who feel that they are the keepers of truth manipulate us in the way that they are doing now ... We must no longer believe in an AIDS virus that supposedly has magic powers, that mutates, that every time they use a new anti-retroviral the virus uses its magic powers to resist."

4. Gudrun Greunke, journalist (Reuters, Spiegel, Stern, ITV), author of several books on scientific and medical controversies, Germany/Spain (jwg00001@teleline.es). "The case that I am going to describe is not directly related to AIDS, but I believe it is the beginning of a pattern, an example of how they manipulate a disease, as they have with AIDS. The issue concerns the Oil Toxic Syndrome, which surprisingly started at the same time as AIDS, 1982. In a family a boy gets sick and is taken to hospital, then three more members of the family become ill and, in the medical records of the emergency room, it is recorded that they all have pneumonia. A physician starts to investigate. Then come more and more similar cases. The media only finds out about it a week later. The physician explains to the relatives that he needs their help since everything indicates that there is a food poisoning. After half an hour of searching it is found that the common food was salad ... Dr. Muro displayed proofs that indicated that the agent responsible for this poisoning was a pesticide from Bayer, but the health authorities in Spain called and gave the case to the CDC. Dr. Muro was fired as Director of Hospital del Rey and officials from the CDC checked his documents and proofs. The official view is that the agent responsible for this poisoning was spoiled olive oil. Up to this date, any alternative view has suffered tremendous censorship from the big media and the scientific journals ...When I see and hear all these discussions about AIDS, I very much remember the case of this oil."

5. Angel Galeano, writer & journalist, author of several books, Director of the newspaper El Pequeño Periódico and of the NGO Fundación Arte y Ciencia, Colombia (Arteyciencia2001@hotmail.com). He presented a brief abstract of the Colombian situation in the time that El Pequeño Periódico was born, 20 years ago in Magangué, a remote and selvatic region of Northern Colombia. He described the tasks of El Centro Médico de Especialistas, directed by Dr Roberto Giraldo, in that region, and the work that they did with cooperatives of peasants and miners. His newspaper helped bring the "Brigades of Health" to distant places in the South of Bolivar, Colombia. He explained that they were forced to leave this region by the guerillas. He also described the role of his newspaper in spreading Giraldo's critical papers on AIDS. The newspaper has published several articles and interviews with various dissident scientists in the last 7 years. The Science and Art Foundation published Dr. Giraldo's first book, AIDS and Stressors. In Colombia, El Pequeño Periódico is the only media outlet that has continued publishing dissident views on AIDS. Galeano proposed the creation of a network of alternative media that would facilitate bringing this information to a wider public.

6. Martin Walker, journalist/researcher (Continuum, The Ecologist), author of Dirty Medicine, England. He read a report that he wrote about "a British family," pointing out that "the ideas that are of interest to the state must be kept under control and that the ideas of medicine are no exception."

He explained that even though it sounded futuristic, we are already living in a world where science and medicine more and more use the legal system as a means to validate their ideas ... "Nothing illustrated better the legal control of medicine than the compulsory treatments and techniques regarding HIV and AIDS." He told the story of an HIV-positive couple, friends of his, and their baby girl, as a way of showing that orthodox medicine and the governments of England and Australia manipulated the law in order to impose upon this couple the prevailing view on AIDS.

7. Montse Arias, journalist, Director of the Spanish version of the journal The Ecologist and of the newsletter Vida Sana, press reporter of Biocultura, Spain (Prensa@vidasana.org). She explained that a powerful censorship is used against the AIDS dissident movement. The fact that there are many newspapers, as is the case in Spain, does not mean that there is democracy. On the contrary, seeing what gets published in the media, the existence of all these media is actually very dangerous, giving the false impression that they are providing varying information and different points of view, while fundamentally they are all official media. She pointed out the case of the newspaper El País. She said that we need to promote the creation of more alternative magazines and newspapers, in order to resist the big media and as a means of bringing to readers other viewpoints, not only on AIDS but on all subjects. She described her very positive experience as Director of The Ecologist in Spanish. She suggested that dissidence is in fact "resistance", and that she would prefer to use this word.

Conclusions of the Round Table with the journalists:
1. All the journalists who attended agreed with the creation of an international network to improve information to the public.

2. In the same manner, we will exchange more documentation from AIDS dissident scientists and circulate this information to journalists in our countries, as a means of breaking the censorship against alternative views on AIDS as well as alternatives on other health and science issues.

3. We promise to exert our efforts to bring together more journalists, editors, TV and radio producers, writers, and directors of the media to convince them to report more extensively on alternative non-toxic treatments for the prevention and healing of AIDS. We need to report specific stories on people with AIDS who have been cured with natural therapies.

4. It was agreed that an example to be followed was the work of Joan Shenton during her 15 years of struggle bringing the other side of AIDS to the public. Other examples of commendable work were the journal The Ecologist, El Pequeño Periódico, and the patient work of hundreds of journalists in many countries who are fighting on a daily basis to bring truths about AIDS to the public.

5. To recognize the important work of the magazine Holistic Medicine, from the Spanish Association of Complementary Medicine, coordinated by Alfredo Embid and Amrit Manthan - an international journal of holistic healing, compiled, edited and published by Dr. Leo Rebello from India.

Other conclusions of this meeting:
1. It is important to point out that during presentations and discussions all attendees agreed that the controversy about the causes of and solutions to AIDS has multiple sides and implications; technical, scientific, medical, ethical, moral, legal, social, political, and economic. It was concluded that solutions will arise from continuing the construction of a great international network of associations, institutions, organizations, celebrities, governments, politicians, artists, investigators, scientists, health care workers, religious leaders, prostitutes, homosexuals, journalists, lawyers, mothers, "seropositive" individuals, and all the rich and poor men and women in all corners of the earth who care about the future of humanity and of other species and who want to participate according to their abilities in the various tasks that the circumstances demand.

2. Emphasis was placed upon the importance of continuing to build an international network of institutions, health care professionals, and alternative therapists who prevent and heal AIDS without anti-retrovirals and other toxic medications. It is crucial that they communicate among themselves and exchange documents, knowledge, expertise, and results.

During his stay in Spain, Dr. Roberto Giraldo was invited to give lectures at the Department of Microbiology, School of Medicine, at the University of Granada, and at the School of Medicine at the University of Barcelona. The latter was presented during an International Congress on Cell Nutrition that was part of the Congress for Life (CMV), organized by Plural 21. Both lectures were well received and it is quite probable that these two orthodox institutions will become a new source of AIDS dissidents.

Similarly, Dr. Leo Rebello from Bombay, India also participated in the "official" conference on AIDS, held a Press Conference at the Media Centre on Step Motherly Treatment to Alternative Medicine, interacted with world leaders, distributed his book AIDS AND ALTERNATIVE MEDICINE, read a poem titled "Aids No More" and conducted Meditation programme.

NOTE: The full text of the conferences and discussions will be published in the journal of Complementary/Holistic Medicines. Also, there is a video of the main lectures and discussions. Interested people please contact the Association of Complementary Medicines in Madrid: www.amcmh.org

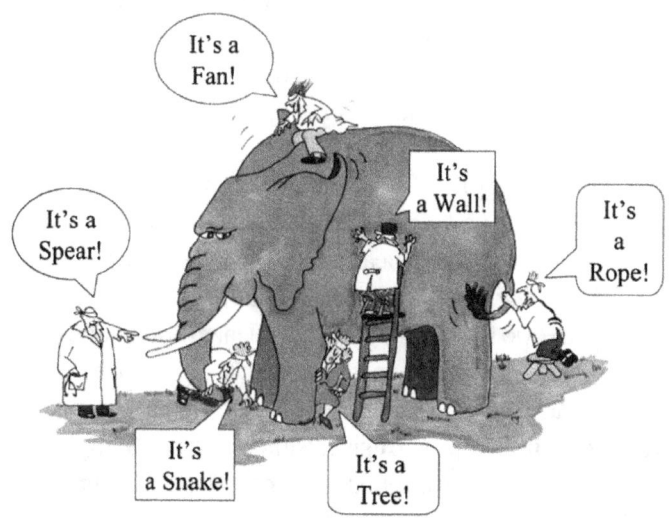

This is how we see the world and then plan. This has to change.
Holistic Healing & Holistic Development for Health & Happiness.

DR. LEO REBELLO REPORT ON XV INTERNATIONAL AIDS CONFERENCE HELD IN BANGKOK, THAILAND, From 11 to 16 July 2004

1.. This was the third consecutive AIDS Conference I attended. The first one was in Durban in 2000 (the best), the second was Barcelona (the worst) and this one, in Bangkok, proved that the Asians have better brains and capacity of organizing, innovation and hospitality. The innovation being the Global Village, which allowed even the school children to visit and learn about this so-called world problem.

2.. 'Global Village' was located strategically on the ground floor in the Impact Convention Center, with the total space of 7,500 m² and was divided conceptually into five zones: Community Radio, Community Market, Spiritual and Mental Health Promotion Centre, Centre for Community Networking and Advocacy and Global Village Coordination Centre. It was for those who could not afford the IAC 2004 registration fee (1000 US dollars) to listen to rubbish like HIV tests, condoms for prevention, carcinogenic anti-retroviral drugs as "life saving" treatment and bogus vaccine trials to hoodwink people.

3. 19,000 delegates from all over the world thronged Bangkok, once infamous for 'free sex' now known for 'safe sex' and 'traditional massage' (foreigners enjoyed it and the locals made brisk business with reasonable rates of 150 Bahts for one hour of therapeutic pressing). Thai hospitality was at its best, exotic food and wine was aplenty (but no one got drunk), fashion clothes much better than in fashion capital France and the goras (whites) went gaga over the chic ethnic couture very affordable. Law and order was excellent, but unobtrusive. Smoking was strictly not allowed inside the conference venue or public transport (luxurious air-conditioned limousine buses).

4. The Thai PM Thaksin Shinawatra, who spoke extempore and delivered a 'politically correct' speech, inaugurated the Conference. UN Secretary-

General Kofi Annan was accompanied by his wife Nane and read out a prepared speech that showed no understanding of the AIDS situation at its best and connivance with the pharma cartel at its worst. The other bigwigs who were present at the AIDS conference included: Nelson Mandela, his second wife Graca Machel, Sonia Gandhi, Miss Universe 2004 Jennifer Hawkins, veteran soul singer Dionne Warwick, Actress Ashley Judd, star of 'Double Jeopardy'; singer Coco Lee, Hollywood star Rupert Everett, the star of movies like 'My Best Friend's Wedding'; Actor and activist Richard Gere (accompanied by Parmeshwar Godrej, Indian socialite), actress-activist Shabana Azmi and hundreds of ministers accustomed to enjoying free trips, roaming aimlessly.

5. I conducted daily workshops at the Global Village on Yoga and Meditation, Naturopathy and Diet for AIDS patients, as also on De-stressing through Drawings and Paintings, which got tremendous response. Thai people at least know about Thai traditional medicine (Ayurveda). As for the mad Americans and Europeans "surviving on mediclaim" less said the better. Their understanding about Holistic Healing modalities is abysmal.

6. XV International AIDS conference, as in the past, began and ended with ARVs, more ARVs and more ARVs. Anti-retroviral drugs (ARVs) offer no cure for AIDS. The toxic effects of ARVs include nerve damage, weakened bones, cancers, unusual accumulation of fat in the neck and abdomen and drug-induced diabetes. Many people have developed dangerously high levels of cholesterol and other lipids in the blood, raising concern that HIV positive persons might face another epidemic of heart disease. Indiscriminate use of ARVs to pregnant mothers is fraught with danger. If a cigarette smoking mother can deliver a 'blue baby', if an alcoholic mother can deliver a 'drunk child', if thalidomide can produce 'monster babies', you are unwittingly playing with the future generation by demanding that the HIV positive mother be given ARVs compulsorily.

7. There are now some 20 ARVs and even if you were to read the mandatory caution, you will wonder how these drugs can be called 'life saving'? But that is how they are promoted and the Africans dance with their 'big botties' and make chimpanzee noises demanding free access to these dangerous drugs, not knowing what the white supremacists are trying to do to them. Their hero Nelson Mandela is unwittingly playing into the hands of Pharma mafia in spreading AIDS SCARE rather than nailing the AIDS LIE. He has formed Nelson Mandela Foundation (NMF) which organised a charity concert in Cape Town in December 2003 (clippings of which were shown on the penultimate day of the conference). Called Campaign 46664, his prison number, to create awareness and fight HIV/AIDS, the politics of NMF are counter to South African President Thabo Mbeiki's sensible policies on HIV/AIDS and malnutrition, the biggest scourge of African continent.

8. Persons Living with AIDS (PLWAs) or the organisers of AIDS conferences (pharma cartel) do not know or pretend not to know that AIDS was started as a population control programme by the CIA. The second phase is to increase the numbers of AIDS patients by false tests designed to test 90% positive and manipulating statistics. Supplying more and more ARVs to larger number of population so that their genes are mutated and the future generations turn out to be zombies, unable to think, oppose or act is the ultimate goal of this sinister programme. AIDS is the biggest con of our times and a few examples will suffice.

9. I asked Dr. Jack Chow, Dy. Director General, WHO: "World Health Assembly has passed several resolutions in favour of integration of traditional and natural medicines for TB and AIDS. Why then the WHO always gives step-motherly treatment to Alternative Medicine in spite of apex body's resolutions? Is that why WHO is now called WHOre of the pharma cartel?". Tongue tied.

10. I asked Prof. Richard Chaisson of John Hopkins: "Your University recently, in association with WHO, declared after extensive study that diet and nutrition can save millions of children from dying. Why then your costly research protocol on the so-called AIDS pandemic has not taken note of this? Is it the case of left hand not knowing what the right hand is doing?". No answer.

11. I asked Dr. Helena Gayle of Gates Foundation and President-elect of

International AIDS Society: "Your foundation has announced another 50 million dollars (chicken feed considering the tax exemption and publicity that Bill Gates will get). But does not even allocate 10% grants to research in traditional and natural medicine. Why? Is it because you know nothing about these systems of medicine or your boss wants to make money now in pharma business having invested heavily in all pharma MNCs?". She was stunned by my straight questions. But being a politician, she said she would discuss them later. Why later? Why not during the IAC when world attention is drawn to it?

12. I persist. I ask them that when V-1 Immunitor (the Thai oral vaccine/nano biotechnology) has shown great efficacy, or when safer homeopathic vaccines (nosodes) are available, why are they not taking it up, they have no answer. I ask them if after 50 years of trials, and billions of dollars down the drain, Cancer vaccine is not found, how can they be so sure that they will be able to find a vaccine against mutating HIV, which itself has not been identified, they gawk at me and take another question. Hundreds of participants look at me with awe or queerly.

13. I personally gave copies of my "AIDS and Alternative Medicine" book (3rd Edition) to (a) Nelson Mandela (b) Sonia Gandhi (c) Richard Gere and several others in the hope that they will get the light of the day. Nelson Mandela, ofcourse, is too old (he is 86) to understand or acknowledge the racket called AIDS. Sonia Gandhi (whose speech was the best and who got a standing ovation for that) did mention en passant about some people not believing in the established theory of AIDS.

14. If only all the above people were to read my foolproof book on AIDS or visited my popular website they will get the complete picture of this so-called AIDS pandemic being drummed up to high crescendo. As Hitler said, "A lie repeated a thousand times becomes truth". Hitler is being blamed for Holocaust (a lie according to some historians), but what about this genocide unleashed by Pharma mafia in the name of AIDS pandemic?

15. For the first time, '2004 AIDS Film Festival' was organised. Held simultaneously at three different venues: **(a)** at Room 11 in Impact Centre **(b)** Lido Cinema and **(c)** Goethe Institut, from 13 to 19 hours, it brought many visitors. 40 Films selected from over 100 received (between April and May 2004) were screened. They dealt with exploitation of women, their low status, the trafficking of young girls, the vast crisis of illiteracy, unemployment, penury and explosive spread of injecting drug use in many countries. Films selected from various geographical regions, themes and genres were in different languages with English sub-titles or voice-overs. I saw one very poignant film titled Meddah (Mercy). It revolves around Luk Nam, an 11-year old girl in Thailand whose life has forever been changed by AIDS. Filmed over two years at a community hospice in the slums of Bangkok, the story unfolds through Luk Nam's diary as she recalls the loss of her family and her best friend.

16. I made the following comments at the end of the film. I am standing here in four capacities: **(a)** as a Parent **(b)** as a Physician **(c)** as a Human Rights Activist and **(d)** as a Communicator. As a Communicator I say that the film is excellent / heart rending. As a Physician (of 25 years standing) I must caution you that the children dying in the community hospice, as is evident from the film, were all dying by drugs, not by disease. Drug reaction and suffering due to them is evident. If only the children could speak and assert, the story would be different. As a Human Rights Activist and Parent, therefore, I shall stand up and speak fearlessly. And my indictment is pharma mafia is killing the children. We are also killing our children either due to ignorance, complicity or silence. After seeing this film I am more convinced that I will have to speak up more fearlessly to stop this sinister game. This report proves the point.

17. I shall conclude this report with two Anecdotes: All the participants at the AIDS conference were given free condoms daily. So, when I received my 100th condom as gift (in less than a week) at the hands of a beautiful, buxom college girl working as a volunteer (there were hundreds of them) I asked her teasingly, "what am I supposed to do with it?". She replied, like a parrot, "use it for safe sex". I retorted, "You have provided a condom, the next logical step is to gift a woman". She blushed, giggled, bowed and answered smartly that her job was only to distribute condoms.

18. At a stall on female condoms, I found a high ranking Thai bureaucrat being 'educated' by the college kids on the benefits of Female condom, and the press personnel going crazy to get that byte. I asked the volunteers at that stall: "Condoms come in how many sizes because African, American women are too big, whereas Thai women are very slim and small". The boys could not answer. I asked the Thai official whether he knew that Penises came in three sizes – 5 inches (standard size), 7 inches and 9 inches (according to Playboy magazine world survey), the official laughed and sneaked away before I could ask him another difficult question.

19. This condom approach (incidentally a condom protects only 60%) is creating condom culture of promiscuity, condom ethics, condom morals, condom generation and condom civilisation. We are writing condomised history. Infact one lady has even created condom wedding gowns and fancy dresses, which you can wear only once like the condoms. If this madness were to continue, there would be only one-night stands, no marriages, and no population on earth. Only selected members of Masonic Mafia, who is masterminding the world, will rule to glory.

20. When AIDS Conference next comes to India in 2010 (proposed), I shall be the first one to organise a parallel conference on AIDS and Alternative Medicine. Let us start preparing from right now to end this AIDS racket which is playing havoc with people's health and lives.

PS: It is now 2014... The proposed AIDS conference has still not come to India. Because we have AYUSH to deal with AIDS.

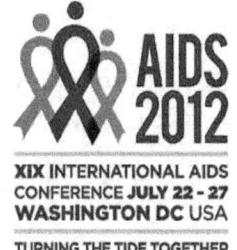

I did not attend this conference eventhough I had the invitation. Because, in USA it is totally drug-based approach, with which I don't agree.

APPRECIATION

—— **Original Message** ——
From: <Cgeshekter@aol.com> To: <leorebello@vsnl.com>
Sent: Friday, May 31, 2002 11:52 AM Subject: Re: It is a shame

Dear Leo:
Good luck with your heroic efforts. I would guess that things at Barcelona will be no different than those at Durban or Vancouver. Only the correct line of thinking will be allowed in the hall; dissenters and critics need not apply. That is exactly how they have run these foolish conferences in the past. A complete farce and travesty...
Best regards,
Charles
Dr. Charles Geshekter, Professor of History, three-time Fulbright Scholar, was the Adviser to US State Department.

—— **Original Message** ——
From: Kola Office To: Dr. Leo Rebello
Sent: Friday, June 28, 2002 6:02 AM
Subject: Re: For Information and Circulation

Dear Leo Rebello,

Thank you for your prompt response to our call for abstracts and Papers. We appreciate your contribution very much and we request that you continue sending us information we can share in the symposium and even in the IYSCA conference.

And we agree to advocate and promote your Slogans of the New Millennium : 'From Aids Scare to Care', Aids No More', 'Health Care is Self Care', 'Humanism in Health' and 'Health, Peace and Plenty for All'.

Regards,
Wilson Kaikai
Organizing Committee Secretary
Chennai

—— **Original Message** ——-
From: <Samin@yogya.wasantara.net.id> To: 'Dr. Leo Rebello'
<leorebello@vsnl.com> Cc: 'Focalpoint' info@focalpointngo.org
Sent: Thursday, July 04, 2002 7:38 AM Subject: Thank you

Dear Dr. Leo,
We got your message regarding AIDS this morning. I have gone thru it
and found it quite interesting...

Thank you for sharing your thoughts and we will keep the paper as basic
reference for our future work. We will also try to visit your website, and
when further queries are needed, we would appreciate the opportunity to
be in touch directly with you.

Best regards,
Farid
SAMIN, Jl. Nitikan Baru No. 95
Yogyakarta 55162, Indonesia
P.O. BOX. 1230, Yogyakarta, 55012
Phone/Fax. +62 (0)274 381101

—— **Original Message** ——
From: International Academy of Classical Homeopathy
<Academy@Vithoulkas.com>
To: Dr. Leo Rebello <leorebello@vsnl.com>
Sent: Friday, January 01, 2002.
Subject: Re: For information

Dear Dr. Leo Rebello
Thank you for the information concerning the AIDS Conference in Barcelona.
We would like to to publish in our Greek journal some portions of your
report on Aids Conference in Barcelona, is it ok with you? Thank you.

Yours sincerely
George Vithoulkas
Right Livelihood Award Winner
Greece

REFERENCES

1. Nature Cure and Yoga Therapy by Dr. Leo Rebello
2. Panacea for Pain by Dr. Leo Rebello
3. Amrit Manthan by Dr. Leo Rebello
4. Encyclopedia of A to Z Alternative Medicines (being compiled) by Dr. Leo Rebello
5. Essays on Health Administration by Dr. Leo Rebello
6. Holistic Healing in Tropical Diseases by Dr. Leo Rebello
7. Pen Power by Dr. Leo Rebello
8. Free, Fair and Fearless by Dr. Leo Rebello
9. Hunza Health Secrets by Renee Taylor
10. Traditional Medicine and Health Care Coverage, WHO Publication
11. Consultations on AIDS and Traditional Medicine, WHO Publication
12. Quarterly Bulletin of CCRH – Vol.15 (3 & 4) 1993
13. Indian Materia Medica in 2 volumes, by Dr. A.K.Nadkarni
14. Agasthia's Herbal Heritage, January 2005
15. National Medicos Medical Journal, October 2002
16. Continuum Magazine, 1998.
17. HIV does not cause AIDS by Dr. Mohammed Ali Al-Bayati, 1999.

WEBSITES :
www.healthwisdom.org
www.virusmyth.net
www.vaclib.org
www.healthfree.org
www.botanicals.net
www.toxi-health.com
www.amcmh.org

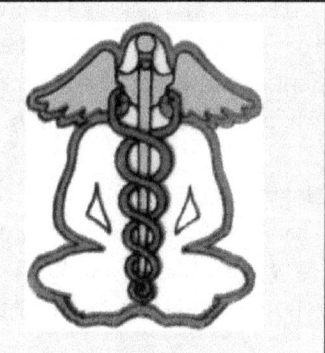

Some pictures are from the internet.

REVISED OATH FOR DOCTORS

© Written and Administered by Dr. Leo Rebello, since 2003

This more comprehensive Oath was drawn by **Dr. Leo Rebello** in 2003, since Hippocrates Oath is now partly outdated being centuries old. This revised Oath has been widely circulated, accepted and appreciated.

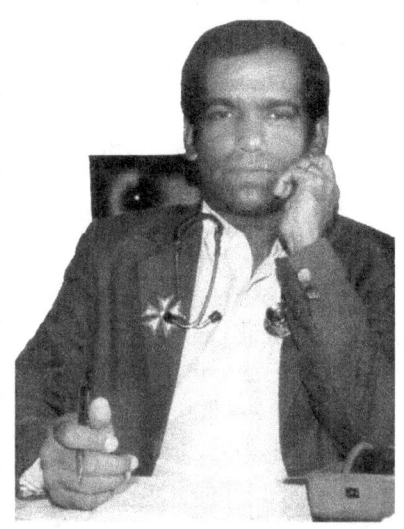

1st July is celebrated as Doctors' Day all over the world. The day usually passes without a whimper. Many doctors have forgotten their Hippocratic oath or humanism. Therefore, I would like to administer the following oath to the doctors to serve as a reminder as to how important is their profession. Doctors to please repeat after me.

I, —————————, do hereby swear on this solemn day that :-
* I shall not prescribe unnecessary medicines and tests to my patients;
* I shall not give false counseling;
* I shall not overcharge and accept cuts and gifts;
* I shall not rape tiny tots with mercury laced innoculations or vaccinations, for they pollute the blood stream leading to serious diseases like AIDS, Cancers, Autism, etc;
* I shall not prescribe lethal drugs, like anti-retrovirals, chemotherapy, or give ECT to my patients;
* I shall not indulge in human organ thefts to the detriment of my patients;
* I shall not be afraid of any authority and fabricate medical records or give false evidence;
* I shall not exploit students studying under me;
* I shall not manipulate findings or results to win grants

I, ——————, further solemnly affirm that:-

* If I cannot treat a disease, I shall not say that AIDS, cancers, diabetes has no cure. But will tell the patient to try other systems of medicine.

* I shall treat health practitioners of other systems with respect and not tell deliberate lies to prove my importance.

* I shall study Holistic healing modalities to increase my knowledge and wisdom.

* I shall not even by mistake say that "HIV=AIDS=Death" or cancers cannot be treated.

* I shall not frighten my patients with unnecessary comments, opinions or advice.

* I still remember what Hippocrates said, namely, "Let diet be your medicine" and shall accordingly prescribe fresh fruits, vegetables and good diet to my patients, rather than tonics, syrups, synthetic multi-vitamins, especially to children.

* I shall not perform surgery, unless it is absolutely must and will not indulge in rackets like amniocentesis, caesarian section, silicon implant or liposuction.

* I shall work to ban the useless and cruel animal experiments in the name of medicine.

* I shall participate in periodic workshops, seminars, conferences at my expense or on scholarship (no pharma funding) to educate myself and speak from my conscience if I am called upon to speak or preside.

* Finally, I shall not consume alcohol, smoke tobacco, or take other narcotic and psychtropic substances. As far as possible, I shall also not take animal proteins.

I realize and aver that a great responsibility of people's well-being is upon my shoulders and I shall carry on my onerous task with utmost dedication.

This I swear in the name of God on this solemn Doctors' Day and I shall repeat this oath daily lest I forget that I am in a divine profession to heal the world.

THE LAST WORD
BURY HIV-AIDS HOAX FIVE-FATHOM DEEP

"The great HIV/AIDS lie was created by Dr. Robert Gallo who was found guilty of 'scientific misconduct'. Instead of trying to prove his insane theories about AIDS to his peers, he went public. Then, with the help of Margaret Heckler, former head of Health and Human Services, who was under great political pressure to come up with an answer to AIDS, the infamous world press announcement of the discovery of the so-called AIDS virus came about. This great fraud is now responsible for the deaths of millions. It was no accident that Gallo just happened to patent the test for HIV the day after the announcement. Gallo is now a multi-millionaire because of AIDS and his fraudulent AIDS test"- Dr. Robert Willner.

The mythical "HIV-induced AIDS plague" in the Third World generates huge sums of cash from Western relief organisations whilst smokescreening the vaccine/drug boys responsible for the carnage.

Glaxo Wellcome's lethal drug, AZT, in combination with the diagnosis of HIV+ and the prediction, stated or implied, that "You will die of AIDS" is one of the worst examples of Medical Black Magic. Millions have been killed on the basis of the ludicrous diagnosis.

Pregnant women who are HIV+ have been told to stop breast-feeding, dosed with AZT, have had abortions or been sterilised. HIV+ babies who become ill - from vaccination and drugs - are automatically diagnosed as "suffering from AIDS". If a caring mother refuses to give the lethal medicine to the child, mother is jailed and the child is taken away to the child care centre by the AIDS Police.

"Considering that there is little scientific proof of the exact linkage of HIV and AIDS, is it ethical to prescribe AZT, a toxic chain terminator of DNA to 150,000 Americans - among them pregnant women and newborn babies.." asked **Rep.G Gutknecht** of the US House of Representatives in March 1995.

AZT began as a "cancer drug" in 1964 but was withdrawn for being too toxic. Its effects include - cancer, hepatitis, dementia, seizures, anxiety, impotence, leukopaenia, severe nausea, ataxia, and the termination of DNA synthesis. AZT eventually kills all those who continue to take it.

"Warning: Retrovir (AZT)...has been associated with symptomatic myopathy, similar to that produced by Human Immunodeficiency Virus" - Glaxo Wellcome literature confirms. None of which, however, stops the medical trade from pushing it on every 'Simple Simon' who is not ill to start with but is labelled as HIV+ and then destroyed by AZT; with AIDS getting the blame - and more billions pouring in for the drug boys, vivisectors, animal breeders and the rest. Now the craze is to give costly, carcinogenic 'cocktail of drugs' to all homosexual men, to poor Africans and Asians, who are "HIV Positive" and "whose numbers are growing". Label them and kill them, to reduce the population of "useless eaters", is the strategy of the neo cons.

A particularly good scam is to haul into court someone "guilty of deliberately infecting the victim with HIV which then develops into full-blown AIDS" - no mention of lethal effect of vaccines, antibiotic damage or carcinogenic AZT. Over 2000 of the world's scientists are now disputing the HIV hoax, their efforts being continually suppressed by the AIDS establishment, the pharmaceutical/vivisection syndicate and their political and media lackeys.

"Regarding the only type of HIV antibody test routinely used since 1992, called an ELISA, manufacturers, Abbott Laboratories, say: 'ELISA testing alone cannot be used to diagnose AIDS". Roche Diagnostics likewise say of their genetic 'HIV testing kits' : "The Amplicor HIV Monitor test is not intended to be used as a screening test for HIV or as a diagnostic test to confirm the presence of HIV infection". "Positive tests do not prove AIDS or pre-AIDS disease status nor that these diseases will be acquired." Manufacturers of Western Blot (HIV) test kit.

"In the general population, which the CDC estimates to have a prevalence of HIV infection of 0.006%, using a test with a specificity of 99%, the result is that 94% of all positives will be false positives." Christine Johnson, Continuum Magazine, April 1994.

"A study done in October 1994 by Congress's Office of Technology Assessment, found that HIV tests can be very inaccurate indeed - 9 in 10 positive findings are called false positives, indicating infection where none exists." US News and World Report, November 23, 1994.

We have all seen them. Stars, disc jockeys, sportsmen and women with a red ribbon pinned onto white tuxedos, black dinner jackets and spaghetti-strapped evening dresses. These are the compassionate celebrities who, with a sad expression, don the mantle of corporate grief for 'AIDS victims and sufferers' and feel they are 'doing good'. Granted they are doing this with the best of intentions but far from doing good they are actually doing damage - they are using their celebrity status to raise funds for AIDS research that is entirely misdirected and orchestrated by a profit-oriented and commercially-blinkered pharmaceutical industry. They are perpetrating the myth of the ... friend who was unlucky enough to get AIDS through one unfortunate sexual encounter. They are diverting attention away from the high-risk lifestyle factors including recreational and intravenous drug use that accompany 'acquired immune deficiency'....

To add to the lunacy, if the HIV existed, a 'positive' response would mean that the body has superiority over the virus. Taking the 'HIV test' is of no use whatsoever to anyone other than drug companies and governments ever eager to increase their control. Those who have had their immune system damaged by vaccines, antibiotics, antipyretics, analgesics, amyl nitrates etc. need to detoxify and to build up immune strength with raw, vegan, organic foods, homeopathic and herbal remedies : and, above all else, to stop swallowing the lethal AZT 'medication'.

The incidence of sickness is growing exceedingly high and a vast number of people live through a lifetime of low and indifferent health. This is because more and more people depend on drugs, as also due to the pollution in the food we eat, the water we drink, the air we breathe, the thoughts we ingest.

Much of this scourge can be avoided by widespread education of the people about the simple principles and methods of health maintenance and a general enlightenment of the public with regard to the lines and techniques of treatment which have yielded the best results.

If you have read this complete book on AIDS thoroughly, you are now ready not only to provide relief for yourself, your near and dear ones, but also to the community at large. We require more Truth Teachers than tongue-tied diplomats, more Health Workers than the fleecing specialists (who know more and more of less and less) and their five star hospitals. If you value your health and the health of your fellowmen, then put your trust in the harmless, effective, economic Alternative Medicine.

The possibilities for healing in Alternative Medicine are immense, the damage zero and the cost insignificant, as compared to the iatrogenesis and frightening costs of treatment of technological medicine. Let us, therefore, demand that atleast 25% of the research funds are allocated to Alternative Medicine and all hospitals have full-fledged AM departments and Medicare also covers AM. Let it be noted that the patients have various rights, like: the right to health, the right to question, the right to choose, the right to know as to why all funds earmarked for health are given only to pseudo-science called modern medicine when we have several proven indigenous systems of medicine. Therein lies the hope for mankind against diseases and suffering.

In conclusion, Adolph Hitler's old adage, "Tell a lie loud enough, and long enough, and the masses will believe it," holds very true when it comes to HIV/AIDS. At least Hitler spoke openly of the truth just as Louis Pasteur on his death bed also finally confessed: "it is not the germ, it is the terrain". However some of those who might blame Hitler for the Holocaust would not have the decency to own up to having killed millions in the name of AIDS cures, cancer treatments or toxic vaccines and thereby unwittingly participating in the insidious Population Control Pogrom eluded to in the 'Useless Eaters' doctrine of the Neo Cons.

QUOTES ONAID$ $CARE

"HIV=AIDS=DEATH is the biggest con perpetrated by the pharma mafia due to which millions have died in the last 25 years. AIDS is not a Science. It is a religious discourse. It is time we stood up against this medical madness. For Silence=Death - of people of ideas and progress". **Dr. Leo Rebello**, President, AIDS Alternativa, Bombay, in a statement issued on July 1, 2006.

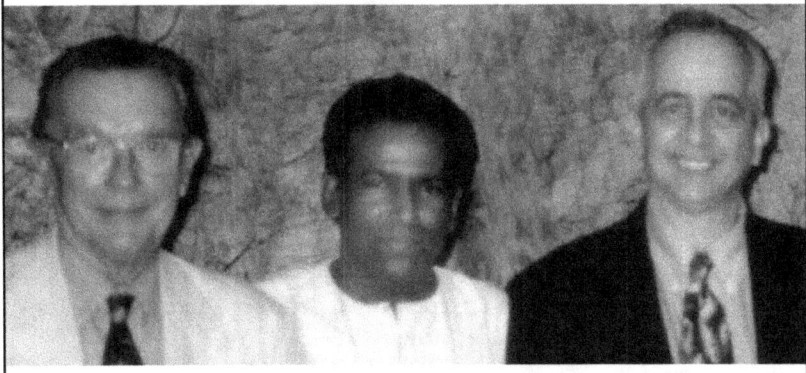

Dr. Etienne de Harven (Canada), Dr. Leo Rebello (India) and Dr. Roberto Giraldo (USA), at the International Conference on Validity of HIV/AIDS Program, Nagpur (India) 30-31 January 2000.

"Dominated by the media, by special pressure groups and by the interests of several pharmaceutical companies, the AIDS establishment's efforts to control the disease lost contact with open-minded, peer-reviewed medical science since the unproven HIV/AIDS hypothesis received 100% of the research funds while all other hypotheses were ignored"... **Dr. Etienne de Harven,** Emeritus Professor of Pathology, at the University of Toronto : Reappraising AIDS / Dec. 1998.

"If there is evidence that HIV causes AIDS, there should be scientific documents which either singly or collectively demonstrate that fact, at least with a high probability. There is no such document." **Dr. Kary Mullis,** Nobel Prize for Chemistry, in Sunday Times, London, 28 Nov. 1993.

"If you think a virus is the cause of AIDS, do a control without it....it hasn't been done. The epidemiology of AIDS is a pile of anecdotal stories, selected to fit the virus/AIDS hypothesis". **Dr. Peter Duesberg,** Member, National Academy of Sciences, who was earlier nominated for Nobel in Medicine and now hounded.

"I have seen the constant terror and the programming to get sick and die...As long as we imply that AIDS exists we are operating within the AIDS group fantasy." **Dr. Michael Ellner,** medical hypnotist.

"Jesus Christ was crucified once. AIDS patients are killed thrice over: **(a)** by disease, scare and ostracism; **(b)** by toxic chemicals; **(c)** by the frightening costs of AIDS medicines. Nobody talks of age-old Holistic Healing. There is more *'Aids Scare'* than *'Aids Care'*.... There is nothing to prove that AIDS is a contagious disease. You cannot get it from anyone. You cannot give it to anyone.... Love is the only contagious disease. Spread the contagion widely for the world needs it desperately". **Dr. Leo Rebello,** at the Traditional Healers March during the XIII International AIDS Conference, Durban, South Africa, July 2000.

"I have known so many people who have died of AIDS... and all of them took the drugs they were told to by their doctors. I have never taken any of them and I haven't gotten sick. Not even a cold. The doctors told me (in 1993) I had 5 years left to live. I am still living. If I had opted for drugs, I would be dead". **Goldie Glitters.**

"I do not regard the causal relationship between HIV and any disease as settled. I have seen considerable evidence that highly improper statistics concerning HIV and AIDS have been passed off as science, and that top members of the scientific establishment have carelessly, if not irresponsibly, joined the media in spreading misinformation about the nature of AIDS". **Dr. Serge Lang,** Professor of Mathematics, Yale University (Yale Scientific, Fall 1994).

"AIDS is brought on by several simultaneous strains on the immune system - drugs, sexually transmitted diseases, multiple viral infections... this whole heterosexual AIDS thing is a hoax". **Dr. Gordon Stewart,** Professor of Public Health, University of Glasgow (Spin June 1992).

"The marketing of HIV, through press releases and statements, as a killer virus causing AIDS without the need for any other factors, has so distorted research and treatment that it may have caused thousands of people to suffer and die". **Dr. Joseph Sonnabend,** founder of AmFAR - Sunday Times, London, 17 May 1992.

"Dr Robert Willner, inoculated himself with the blood of **Pedro Tocino,** a HIV+ haemophiliac, on live Spanish television in 1993: an event which was not picked up by the pharma-beholden British or US media" - **Patrick Rattigan,** Naturopath, UK.

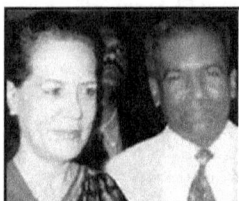 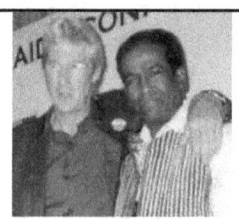 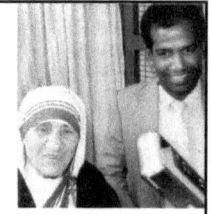

Dr. Leo Rebello with Ms Sonia Gandhi, MP and Actor Richard Gere at the XV International AIDS Conference, Bangkok, in 2004 and with Mother Teresa in December 1989 when he formed AIDS Alternativa.